Ovarian Hyperstimulation Syndrome (OHSS) Free Clinic

Gautam Nand Allahbadia
Akanksha Allahbadia Gupta
Swati Gautam Allahbadia
Editors

Ovarian Hyperstimulation Syndrome (OHSS) Free Clinic

An Algorithm for Change

Springer

Editors
Gautam Nand Allahbadia
Allahbadia Fertility Clinic
Dubai, United Arab Emirates

Akanksha Allahbadia Gupta
Sumitra Hospital
Noida, Uttar Pradesh, India

Swati Gautam Allahbadia
Rotunda – The Center for Human Reproduction
Wadala (West), Mumbai, Maharashtra, India

ISBN 978-981-95-3288-9 ISBN 978-981-95-3289-6 (eBook)
https://doi.org/10.1007/978-981-95-3289-6

This Springer imprint is published by the registered company Springer Nature Singapore Pte Ltd.
The registered company address is: 152 Beach Road, #21-01/04 Gateway East, Singapore 189721, Singapore

Foreword

The landscape of fertility treatment has evolved significantly in recent decades, with breakthroughs in science and technology offering hope to individuals and couples seeking to start a family. In vitro fertilization (IVF) is one such treatment option that has offered hope to millions of patients worldwide. IVF was initially offered by only a few centers and success rates were low. Over the past four decades, IVF has become widely available, and remarkable advances have been made due to which success rates have significantly improved. These advances include better medications being used for controlled ovarian hyperstimulation (COH), stimulation protocols, and laboratory techniques, e.g., intracytoplasmic sperm injection (ICSI), pre-implantation genetic testing (PGT), and embryo transfer technique. Elective single embryo transfer has reduced the incidence of multiple pregnancy which was historically a major problem with IVF. With increasing success rates, the focus has now shifted to IVF safety.

Ovarian hyperstimulation syndrome (OHSS) is a major complication associated with IVF and continues to present significant challenges. According to the Practice Committee of the American Society for Reproductive Medicine, moderate-to-severe OHSS occurs in approximately 1% to 5% of cycles. Typical findings include ovarian enlargement, ascites, hemoconcentration, hypercoagulability, and electrolyte imbalances. Symptoms are often qualified by their severity (mild, moderate, or severe) and by the timing of onset (early or late). Severe OHSS can lead to serious complications, including pleural effusion, acute renal insufficiency, and venous thromboembolism.

Prevention of severe OHSS is of paramount importance during COH. This book, *Ovarian Hyperstimulation-Free Clinic: An Algorithm for Change*, emerges as a timely and essential guide for both medical professionals and patients alike. The authors have crafted a comprehensive resource that not only explores the science behind OHSS but also introduces practical algorithms for implementing systemic change within clinical settings. The goal is clear: to improve outcomes, minimize risks, and offer personalized care that accounts for the unique needs of each patient.

Understanding the pathophysiology of this condition may aid in identifying measures to prevent its development and treat associated symptoms. The proper staging of the disease, prediction and risk factors of OHSS, role of new biochemical markers in its prevention, and role of ultrasound have all been discussed in detail. Individualizing stimulation protocols to prevent OHSS, luteal phase strategies to prevent OHSS, interventional rescue strategies for unexpected OHSS, and role of in vitro maturation (IVM) are some of the topics discussed in this book. Finally, Dr. Allahbadia addresses an important question—"Is there an ideal stimulation protocol for an OHSS-free clinic?"

Dr. Gautam Allahbadia has authored more than a dozen books over the past two decades. Once again, in this book he has compiled the views of a series of international experts in the management of OHSS. In a field where precision and adaptability are paramount, this book provides a roadmap for embracing innovation while keeping patient safety and well-being at the forefront. It challenges outdated methodologies and offers fresh perspectives on how clinics can optimize their approaches through data-driven insights, advanced protocols, and compassionate care.

Whether you are a healthcare provider, a researcher, or someone navigating the journey of fertility treatment, this book will empower you with the knowledge, strategies, and confidence to advocate for and implement meaningful change. The future of fertility care lies not just in technological advancement, but in the thoughtful application of that technology—this book serves as an essential guide to making that future a reality.

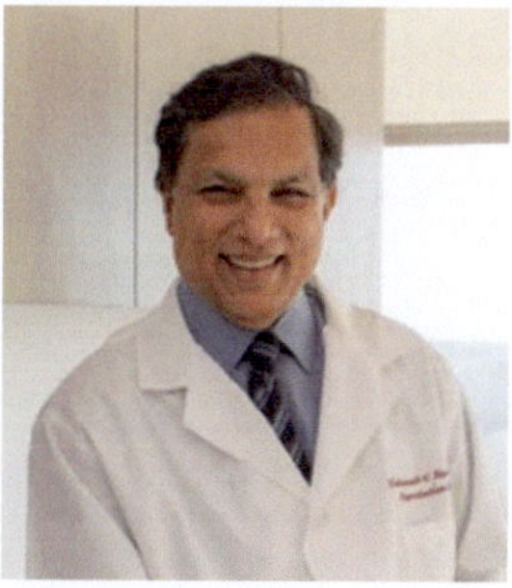

President, Medical Director
Director IVF Program
InVia Fertility Specialists
Hoffman Estates, IL, USA

Vishvanath C. Karande

Contents

About the Editors

Gautam Nand Allahbadia is Consultant Reproductive Endocrinology & IVF at Allahbadia IVF, DHCC; Bourn Hall Fertility Clinic, Dubai; and FertiClinic Fertilization Center, Sharjah, UAE. He is the founder and academic mentor of Rotunda—The Center for Human Reproduction, the world-renowned fertility clinic in Mumbai. He is a noted world authority on Ultrasound-guided Embryo transfers and one of the pioneers in Third Party Reproduction in Southeast Asia. He was responsible for India's first trans-ethnic surrogate pregnancy involving a Chinese couple's baby delivered by an unrelated Indian surrogate mother. He is the Emeritus Editor of the *Journal of Obstetrics & Gynecology* of India as well as the IVF Lite (*Journal of Minimal Stimulation IVF*). He cherishes over 150 peer-reviewed publications, 142 book chapters, and 31 textbooks, the latest being a comprehensive two book set textbook published by Springer International, entitled *Textbook of Assisted Reproduction*, and is on the Editorial Board of several international journals. He was elected as the Vice President of the World Association of Reproductive Medicine (WARM), headquartered in Rome, and "Mumbai's Top Doc" for 2012 by a peer nomination process.

Akanksha Allahbadia Gupta is a Consultant in Infertility and Reproductive Medicine at Indira IVF, Delhi, India, as well as at Sumitra Hospital, Noida, India. She has previously worked at the prestigious Infertility clinic Rotunda—The Center for Human Reproduction in Parel, India. She has worked in Gynecological

Oncology as well as the Women's Health Departments in the Massachusetts General Hospital as part of her training with Harvard Medical School, Boston. She has completed her fellowship in Minimal Access Surgery from the World Laparoscopy Hospital, Gurgaon, India. She is also a certified assessor for ART center accreditation as part of the Quality and Accreditation Institute. She has been involved in over a thousand IVF procedures, managing a variety of cases including patients with high-risk pregnancies, multiple gestations, male factor infertility, endometriosis, multiple fibroids, Mullerian anomalies, premature ovarian failure, and recurrent pregnancy losses. She has won multiple prizes in paper and poster presentations at national level. She is also a co-author in over 50 manuscripts contributed to internationally acclaimed textbooks and peer-reviewed journals.

Swati Gautam Allahbadia is a leading Fertility Physician, Endoscopist, and Obstetrician based in Mumbai and working in Women's health since the last 30 years. She did her graduate and postgraduate studies in Medicine and Gynecology from the Seth G S Medical College and KEM Hospitals. She was a holder of the V N Majumdar prize in that period. She has been Lecturer, Associate Professor, and Unit Head at a Government Hospital in Mumbai. She trained in Endoscopy at the Ethicon Institute and as a holder of the Hargobind Fellowship, trained in Endoscopic microsurgery as well as Robotic Surgery in the United States. She holds Diplomas in Endoscopy and in Reproductive Medicine from Germany.

She currently manages Rotunda—The Center for Human Reproduction, Wadala, Mumbai, and has helped patients from India and across the globe achieve their dream of completing their families. At Rotunda, she has managed several cases including patients with multiple IVF failures, endometriosis, ovarian tumors, diminished ovarian reserve, and recurrent pregnancy losses.

She is attached to the Global, Raheja, Breach Candy, and Wadia hospitals in Mumbai. You can read more about her work at www.swatiallahbadia.com.

Pathophysiology of OHSS: Is It Always Iatrogenic?

1

Gil Gutvirtz and Eitan Lunenfeld

1.1 Introduction

In a natural ovulatory cycle, hypothalamic-pituitary-ovarian feedback mechanisms restrict follicular recruitment to a limited number of early antral follicles. From these, a single dominant follicle is selected to ovulate in response to a marked rise in serum luteinizing hormone (LH), known as the "LH surge." Prior to oocyte release, LH leads to the luteinization of the granulosa cells surrounding the oocyte. Following ovulation, the remaining follicle, known as the corpus luteum, secretes both progesterone, estradiol, and inhibin A. Progesterone secretion by the corpus luteum plays a vital role in sustaining the uterine endometrial lining, which is essential for embryo implantation and subsequent development. In the absence of implantation, the corpus luteum will

G. Gutvirtz
Soroka University Medical Center, Beer-Sheva, Israel

Faculty of Health Sciences, Ben-Gurion University of the Negev, Beer-Sheva, Israel

E. Lunenfeld (✉)
Faculty of Health Sciences, Ben-Gurion University of the Negev, Beer-Sheva, Israel

Adelson School of Medicine, Ariel University, Ariel, Israel

G. N. Allahbadia et al. (eds.), *Ovarian Hyperstimulation Syndrome (OHSS) Free Clinic*, https://doi.org/10.1007/978-981-95-3289-6_1

regress, progesterone secretion will decay over time, and the corpus luteum will turn into a corpus albicans. Without progesterone maintaining the endometrium, the endometrial lining will shed, resulting in menstruation.

However, if implantation occurs, the syncytiotrophoblast cells of the developing embryo will secrete human chorionic gonadotropin (hCG), which is vital for corpus luteum survival and the continuation of progesterone and estrogen secretion.

Remarkably, the mature corpus luteum has the highest blood flow per unit of tissue of any organ in the body [1, 2]. Consequently, angiogenesis is a critical component of its development, driven by key angiogenic growth factors such as vascular endothelial growth factor (VEGF) [3].

1.2 Ovarian Hyperstimulation Syndrome (OHSS)

Ovarian hyperstimulation syndrome (OHSS) represents the most severe complication of controlled ovarian hyperstimulation (COH) and can be viewed as an exaggeration of a physiologic process. In the setting of ovarian stimulation for ART, gonadotropin administration overrides the normal FSH threshold and feedback mechanisms, in a normal ovulating menstrual cycle are designed for mono-follicular development, resulting in multiple folliculogenesis.

Women affected by OHSS typically present with enlarged ovaries and markedly increased vascular permeability, leading to significant fluid shifts and accumulation within the peritoneal cavity—an effect almost invariably triggered by the administration of human chorionic gonadotropin (hCG) [4]. Severe OHSS may also manifest with hypovolemia, oliguria progressing to renal impairment, pleural effusion or hydrothorax, hemoconcentration, and thromboembolic events, which in rare cases can be life-threatening.

The recruitment of a substantial number of small antral follicles into a functional cohort leads to the formation of multiple large antral follicles, which, when triggered to ovulate, produce excessive amounts of VEGF by the developing corpus luteum.

The vascular endothelial growth factor (VEGF) family comprises key physiological regulators of angiogenesis and mediators of vascular endothelial permeability [5]. Among its members, VEGF-A plays a central role in ovarian angiogenesis, promoting normal follicular development and supporting corpus luteum function [6, 7]. Excessive VEGF production leads to exaggerated perifollicular neovascularization. The newly formed blood vessels exhibit increased permeability, which facilitates the leakage of follicular and perifollicular fluid containing large amounts of VEGF into the peritoneal cavity. This process is followed by functional impairment of blood vessels in the ovaries and peritoneal cavity, which leads to massive fluid shift from the intravascular space to the third compartment, also known as the "third spacing," resulting in intravascular hypovolemia concomitant with fluid accumulation in tissues (abdomen, thorax, pericardium, etc.). Studies in both humans and rodents have indicated that the VEGF/VEGFR2 signaling pathway mediates increased vascular permeability, which is primarily responsible for the significant fluid shift from the intravascular space into the peritoneal cavity [8].

Although the most severe form of OHSS is rare nowadays, it has a potentially fatal outcome if impaired cardiac, renal, pulmonary, and liver function leads to organ failure.

A key element in the pathogenesis of OHSS is the use of human chorionic gonadotropin (hCG) to trigger ovulation. OHSS rarely develops in the absence of an ovulatory dose of hCG [9, 10]. Exogenous hCG triggers extensive luteinization of granulosa cells, a key step in the pathogenesis of OHSS. This risk may be mitigated by using alternative agents, such as gonadotropin-releasing hormone (GnRH) agonists, to induce final oocyte maturation [11].

The potent effect of hCG is attributed to its higher dosage and prolonged half-life, resulting in biological activity that is six to seven times greater than that of endogenous luteinizing hormone (LH) [12].

The successive stages of OHSS are summarized in Fig. 1.1.

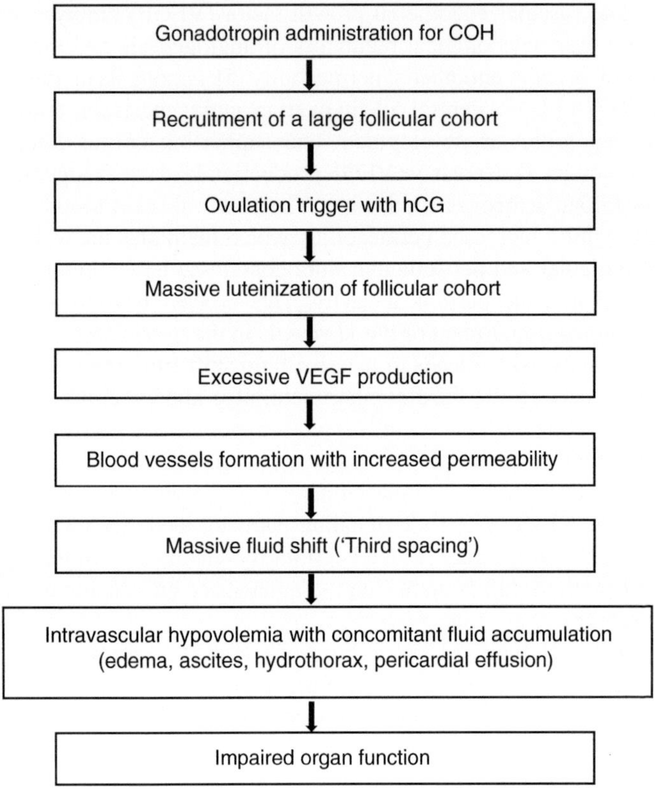

Fig. 1.1 Pathogenesis of iatrogenic OHSS

1.3 Spontaneous OHSS

OHSS is almost exclusively an iatrogenic complication of controlled ovarian hyperstimulation (COH) using exogenous hCG. However, rare cases of spontaneous OHSS have been described in the literature over the years; most reports included late OHSS in women who have spontaneously conceived [13, 14], specifically those with abnormally high levels of endogenous hCG as seen in multiple pregnancies [15–17] or molar pregnancies [18–20]. In some instances, OHSS may result from elevated levels of endogenous gonadotropin-like hormones, such as thyroid-stimulating hormone (TSH) [21], or from increased ovarian sensitivity to endogenous gonadotropins, often due to mutations in the follicle-stimulating hormone (FSH) receptor [22].

In their work from 2006, De Leener et al. [23] suggested a classification system of spontaneous OHSS, including three types: **Type I** consists of pregnant patients in the first trimester who presented with normal hCG levels but were found to have mutations in the FSH receptor, leading to enhanced sensitivity to endogenous gonadotropins. So far, at least six pathogenic heterozygous FSHR mutations have been described in patients with spontaneous OHSS [24]. **Type II** consists of pregnant patients with OHSS secondary to elevated levels of hCG seen in hydatidiform mole or multiple pregnancies. **Type III** consists of nonpregnant patients with OHSS due to primary (usually long-standing) hypothyroidism.

While most cases of spontaneous OHSS fall into one of these categories, Panagiotopoulou et al. [24] claim that this classification, however, fails to describe cases of spontaneous OHSS secondary to high FSH or LH levels. They therefore proposed a revision to the De Leener classification by introducing a fourth type—**type IV**—characterized by gonadotrophin-secreting adenomas producing FSH or LH.

Whatever the underlying etiology for spontaneous OHSS, it appears that the interaction between glycoprotein hormones (hCG, TSH, FSH, and LH) and the FSH receptor is the prerequisite for the development of spontaneous OHSS. Glycoprotein hormones are heterodimeric molecules composed of a shared α-subunit and a unique β-subunit that confers receptor specificity. Their receptors belong to the G-protein-coupled receptor family and are distinguished by a large extracellular domain that facilitates specific hormone recognition and binding. It has been proposed that structural similarities in the β-subunits of the four glycoprotein hormones may allow for cross-activation of the FSH receptor. Additionally, elevated levels of these hormones may surpass receptor specificity, leading to unintended receptor activation

[25]. Analogous to TSH receptor mutations that increase affinity for hCG—as implicated in gestational hyperthyroidism [26]—mutations in the FSH receptor can reduce ligand specificity, enabling activation of the mutated receptor by hCG [27]. Mutations in the FSH receptor (FSHR) may be activating, predisposing individuals to OHSS, or inactivating, leading to infertility due to an inadequate ovarian response to gonadotropins. To date, six pathogenic heterozygous activating FSHR mutations have been identified in patients with spontaneous OHSS [24]. The mutated FSH receptors exhibit heightened sensitivity to hCG, resulting in inappropriate activation by hCG and subsequent development of OHSS. In contrast, activating FSHR mutations have not been identified in women with iatrogenic OHSS [28]. A single case report suggested a possible mutation in the LH receptor gene in a patient with spontaneous OHSS, though this finding remains unconfirmed [29].

This hypothesis may also explain the difference in the timing at which spontaneous OHSS occurs. While iatrogenic OHSS usually develops soon after hCG administration, spontaneous cases of OHSS related to pregnancy appear in the late first trimester (between 8 and 12 weeks) when gestational hCG peaks [30]. As explained by Delbaere et al., "That is because in the iatrogenic form, the follicular recruitment and enlargement occur during ovarian stimulation with exogenous FSH, while in the spontaneous form, the follicular recruitment occurs later through the stimulation of the FSH receptor by pregnancy-derived hCG. However, in both forms, massive luteinization of enlarged stimulated ovaries ensues, inducing the release of vasoactive mediators, leading to the development of the symptoms of OHSS."

1.4 Conclusion

OHSS is mostly iatrogenic and could be predicted during ovarian stimulation in women with risk factors. Hence, preventive measures should be taken to avoid iatrogenic OHSS.

However, spontaneous OHSS is almost always unpredictable, and most clinicians have low suspicion of OHSS in women who are not undergoing fertility treatments. In some cases, it may be mistaken for an ovarian tumor due to similar features such as abdominal distension, ascites, and enlarged ovaries. This chapter describes the pathophysiology of OHSS and highlights cases of spontaneous forms of OHSS in order to alert clinicians regarding this rare but potentially life-threatening entity.

References

1. Reynolds LP, Redmer DA. Growth and development of the corpus luteum. J Reprod Fertil Suppl. 1999;54:181–91.
2. Reynolds LP, Grazul-Bilska AT, Redmer DA. Angiogenesis in the corpus luteum. Endocrine. 2000;12(1):1–9. eng
3. Smith MF, McIntush EW, Smith GW. Mechanisms associated with corpus luteum development. J Anim Sci. 1994;72(7):1857–72. eng
4. Kumar P, Sait SF, Sharma A, Kumar M. Ovarian hyperstimulation syndrome. J Hum Reprod Sci. 2011;4(2):70–5. PMCID: PMC3205536. eng
5. Ferrara N, Davis-Smyth T. The biology of vascular endothelial growth factor. Endocr Rev. 1997;18(1):4–25. eng
6. Geva E, Jaffe RB. Role of vascular endothelial growth factor in ovarian physiology and pathology. Fertil Steril. 2000;74(3):429–38.
7. Harada M, Peegel H, Menon KM. Expression of vascular endothelial growth factor a during ligand-induced down-regulation of luteinizing hormone receptor in the ovary. Mol Cell Endocrinol. 2010;328(1–2):28–33. PMCID: PMC2947199. Epub 20100707. eng
8. Zheng C, Gulappa T, Menon B, Menon KMJ. Association between LH receptor regulation and ovarian hyperstimulation syndrome in a rodent model. Reproduction. 2020;160(2):239–45. PMCID: PMC9429945. eng
9. Aboulghar MA, Mansour RT. Ovarian hyperstimulation syndrome: classifications and critical analysis of preventive measures. Hum Reprod Update. 2003;9(3):275–89. eng
10. Schenker JG. Prevention and treatment of ovarian hyperstimulation. Hum Reprod. 1993;8(5):653–9. eng
11. Soares SR, Gómez R, Simón C, García-Velasco JA, Pellicer A. Targeting the vascular endothelial growth factor system to prevent ovarian hyperstimulation syndrome. Hum Reprod Update. 2008;14(4):321–33.
12. Yen SS, Llerena O, Little B, Pearson OH. Disappearance rates of endogenous luteinizing hormone and chorionic gonadotropin in man. J Clin Endocrinol Metab. 1968;28(12):1763–7. eng
13. Foulk RA, Martin MC, Jerkins GL, Laros RK. Hyperreactio luteinalis differentiated from severe ovarian hyperstimulation syndrome in a spon-

taneously conceived pregnancy. Am J Obstet Gynecol. 1997;176(6):1300-2.
14. Schnorr JA, Miller H, Davis JR, Hatch K, Seeds J. Hyperreactio luteinalis associated with pregnancy: a case report and review of the literature. Am J Perinatol. 1996;13(2):95–7. eng
15. Daolio J, Sperduti S, Casarini L, Falbo A, Materazzo C, Aguzzoli L, et al. Spontaneous and iatrogenic ovarian hyperstimulation syndrome in the absence of FSHR mutations: a case report of two unexpected cases. BMC Med Genet. 2023;16(1):45. PMCID: PMC9990314. Epub 20230307. eng
16. Check JH, Choe JK, Nazari A. Hyperreactio luteinalis despite the absence of a corpus luteum and suppressed serum follicle stimulating concentrations in a triplet pregnancy. Hum Reprod. 2000;15(5):1043–5. eng
17. Suzuki S. Comparison between spontaneous ovarian hyperstimulation syndrome and hyperreactio luteinalis. Arch Gynecol Obstet. 2004;269(3):227–9. Epub 20031218. eng
18. Arora R, Merhi ZO, Khulpateea N, Roth D, Minkoff H. Ovarian hyperstimulation syndrome after a molar pregnancy evacuation. Fertil Steril. 2008;90(4):1197.e5–7. Epub 20080114. eng
19. Strafford M, Moreno-Ruiz N, Stubblefield P. Ovarian hyperstimulation syndrome in a spontaneous pregnancy with a complete hydatidiform mole. Fertil Steril. 2009;92(1):395.e1–3. Epub 20090414. eng
20. Zhou X, Duan Z. A case of ovarian hyperstimulation syndrome following a spontaneous complete hydatidiform molar pregnancy. Gynecol Endocrinol. 2012;28(11):850–2. Epub 20120516. eng
21. Edwards-Silva RN, Han CS, Hoang Y, Kao LC. Spontaneous ovarian hyperstimulation in a naturally conceived pregnancy with uncontrolled hypothyroidism. Obstet Gynecol. 2008;111(2 Pt 2):498–501.
22. Vasseur C, Rodien P, Beau I, Desroches A, Gérard C, de Poncheville L, et al. A chorionic gonadotropin-sensitive mutation in the follicle-stimulating hormone receptor as a cause of familial gestational spontaneous ovarian hyperstimulation syndrome. N Engl J Med. 2003;349(8):753–9. eng
23. De Leener A, Montanelli L, Van Durme J, Chae H, Smits G, Vassart G, et al. Presence and absence of follicle-stimulating hormone receptor mutations provide some insights into spontaneous ovarian hyperstimulation syndrome physiopathology. J Clin Endocrinol Metab. 2006;91(2):555–62. Epub 20051108. eng
24. Panagiotopoulou N, Byers H, Newman WG, Bhatia K. Spontaneous ovarian hyperstimulation syndrome: case report, pathophysiological classification and diagnostic algorithm. Eur J Obstet Gynecol Reprod Biol. 2013;169(2):143–8. Epub 20130403. eng
25. Schubert RL, Narayan P, Puett D. Specificity of cognate ligand-receptor interactions: fusion proteins of human chorionic gonadotropin and the heptahelical receptors for human luteinizing hormone, thyroid-stimulat-

ing hormone, and follicle-stimulating hormone. Endocrinology. 2003;144(1):129–37. eng

26. Rodien P, Brémont C, Sanson ML, Parma J, Van Sande J, Costagliola S, et al. Familial gestational hyperthyroidism caused by a mutant thyrotropin receptor hypersensitive to human chorionic gonadotropin. N Engl J Med. 1998;339(25):1823–6. eng
27. Delbaere A, Smits G, Olatunbosun O, Pierson R, Vassart G, Costagliola S. New insights into the pathophysiology of ovarian hyperstimulation syndrome. What makes the difference between spontaneous and iatrogenic syndrome? Hum Reprod. 2004;19(3):486–9. PMCID: PMC2891954. Epub 20040129. eng
28. d'Alva CB, Serafini P, Motta E, Kohek MB, Latronico AC, Mendonca BB. Absence of follicle-stimulating hormone receptor activating mutations in women with iatrogenic ovarian hyperstimulation syndrome. Fertil Steril. 2005;83(6):1695–9. eng
29. Kerkelä E, Skottman H, Friden B, Bjuresten K, Kere J, Hovatta O. Exclusion of coding-region mutations in luteinizing hormone and follicle-stimulating hormone receptor genes as the cause of ovarian hyperstimulation syndrome. Fertil Steril. 2007;87(3):603–6.
30. De Leener A, Caltabiano G, Erkan S, Idil M, Vassart G, Pardo L, et al. Identification of the first germline mutation in the extracellular domain of the follitropin receptor responsible for spontaneous ovarian hyperstimulation syndrome. Hum Mutat. 2008;29(1):91–8. eng

2 Current Concepts, Etiopathology, and Staging of OHSS

Mona Shroff

2.1 Introduction

Ovarian hyperstimulation syndrome (OHSS) is a serious and potentially life-threatening complication that can occur during ovulation stimulation, especially in the context of assisted reproductive technologies (ART). A complex interaction of hormonal, vascular, and genetic elements influences its development. While human chorionic gonadotropin (hCG) is commonly recognised as a primary trigger, emerging evidence indicates that OHSS may occasionally develop even in its absence. The hallmark of this condition is heightened capillary permeability, which results in significant fluid displacement and systemic effects. A clear understanding of the contributing mechanisms is essential for effective prevention and treatment strategies.

M. Shroff (✉)
Nova IVF Fertility, Surat, Gujarat, India

G. N. Allahbadia et al. (eds.), *Ovarian Hyperstimulation Syndrome (OHSS) Free Clinic*, https://doi.org/10.1007/978-981-95-3289-6_2

2.2 Current Concepts in Etiopathogenesis (Table 2.1)

2.2.1 Hormonal Triggers

Human chorionic gonadotropin (hCG): hCG is a critical trigger for OHSS, either administered exogenously for ovulation induction or produced endogenously by the trophoblast during early pregnancy. It induces extensive luteinisation of granulosa cells, stimulating the growth of new ovarian blood vessels and initiating a sequence of events that increase vascular permeability and fluid movement [1]. It is likely an exaggerated response to normal luteinising hormone (LH). This degree of luteinisation is typically absent when alternative agents, such as gonadotropin-releasing hormone (GnRH) agonists, are used for final oocyte maturation. The strong physiological impact of hCG is linked to its much longer half-life and a biological potency that is approximately six to seven times greater than that of natural LH [2].

Table 2.1 Etiopathogenesis of OHSS

Etiopathogenesis
Hormonal triggers
Human chorionic gonadotropin (hCG)
Vascular and cytokine factors
Vascular endothelial growth factor (VEGF)
Cytokines and inflammatory mediators
Angiotensin-renin-aldosterone system
Genetic predisposing factors
Polycystic ovarian syndrome (PCOS)
Follicle-stimulating hormone receptor (FSHR) mutations
Single-nucleotide polymorphisms (SNPs)
Anti-Müllerian hormone (AMH) signalling pathway
Long non-coding RNAs (lncRNAs)
Other genetic variants and signalling pathways
Immune cell involvement and other molecular factors
Exosomal miRNAs
Melatonin and receptor expression
Clinical and demographic factors
Younger age, low BMI, allergies, multiple follicles, high estradiol

2.2.2 Vascular and Cytokine Factors

- *Vascular endothelial growth factor (VEGF):* VEGF, a member of the heparin-binding protein family, acts directly on endothelial cells to stimulate both their growth and the formation of new blood vessels. Its mRNA and protein forms are produced by granulosa and theca cells during the later stages of follicular development and post-ovulation [3]. hCG significantly upregulates its expression and is a pivotal factor in OHSS, promoting increased capillary permeability and neo-angiogenesis in the ovaries. This leads to the characteristic fluid shifts seen in the syndrome [3, 4]. The interaction between VEGF and its receptor VEGFR-2 is crucial. hCG administration leads to increased VEGF and VEGFR-2 mRNA expression, correlating with peak vascular permeability [5, 6]. Although the precise mechanisms by which the VEGF-VEGFR-2 complex enhances vascular permeability remain unclear, it is hypothesised that downstream pathways affecting endothelial cell-to-cell junctions may contribute to this process. The presence of hCG receptors on endothelial cells and the subsequent VEGF release suggest an autocrine-paracrine mechanism that exacerbates the permeability changes characteristic of OHSS. Dopamine agonists like cabergoline have been demonstrated to inhibit VEGFR-2 phosphorylation, offering a preventive strategy for high-risk patients [2, 6].
- *Cytokines and inflammatory mediators:* Several cytokines, such as interleukins (IL-1, IL-2, IL-6, IL-8) and tumour necrosis factor-alpha (TNF-α), play a role in driving the inflammatory processes and vascular alterations that are linked to the development of OHSS [4].
- *Angiotensin-renin-aldosterone system:* The angiotensin-renin-aldosterone system, along with the kinin-kallikrein system, is involved in developing OHSS, with angiotensin II playing a crucial role. This system regulates fluid balance and vascular tone, influencing the severity of OHSS [7].

2.2.3 Genetic Predisposing Factors

- *Polycystic ovarian syndrome (PCOS):* Women diagnosed with PCOS are more susceptible to OHSS, largely because their ovaries respond more intensely to gonadotropin stimulation, and they typically exhibit elevated baseline levels of androgens and oestrogens [1].
- *Genetic variations:* Various genetic polymorphisms and mutations have been identified that contribute to the susceptibility and severity of OHSS. These genetic variations can affect hormone receptors and signalling pathways, influencing ovarian response to stimulation.
- *Follicle-stimulating hormone receptor (FSHR) mutations:* Mutations in the FSH receptor (FSHR) are a well-documented genetic factor in OHSS. These mutations can lead to increased sensitivity to hCG and, in some cases, thyrotropin (TSH), resulting in spontaneous OHSS. Notable mutations include *T449I, D567N,* and *T449A*, which alter the receptor's sensitivity and basal activity, contributing to the syndrome's pathogenesis [8]. The Ser680Asn variation in the *FSHR* gene has been linked to severe OHSS. Specifically, the Ser/Ser genotype shows reduced sensitivity to follicle-stimulating hormone (FSH), which can influence oestradiol levels and the ovarian response [9].
- *Single-nucleotide polymorphisms (SNPs):* Several SNPs have been linked to OHSS, including those in the *MTHFR, AMHR2,* and *LHCGR* genes. As per Ghaderian et al., "The MTHFR rs1801131 C-allele and rs1801133 T-allele, AMHR2 rs2002555 G-allele, and LHCGR rs2293275 G-allele are more prevalent in OHSS patients, suggesting these alleles as independent risk factors for the syndrome. In contrast, the PGR rs10895068 A-allele appears to have a protective effect against OHSS, being more common in individuals with a normal ovarian response" [10].

- *Anti-Müllerian hormone (AMH) signalling pathway:* Although SNPs in the AMH signalling pathway were investigated, no significant association with early OHSS was found in a study involving Han Chinese women. This suggests that while AMH is crucial for ovarian function, its genetic variations may not directly contribute to OHSS in all populations. The SNP rs10407022 was associated with a higher ovarian response, suggesting a potential role in OHSS pathogenesis indirectly through enhanced follicular activity [11].
- *Long non-coding RNAs (lncRNAs):* Differential expression of lncRNAs has been observed in OHSS, with certain lncRNAs being upregulated or downregulated in granulosa cells. These lncRNAs may play roles in the biological processes associated with OHSS, although their exact mechanisms remain to be elucidated [12].
- *Other genetic variants:* Rare genetic variants, such as those in the *FLT4* gene, have been suggested to potentially contribute to OHSS, although further research is needed to confirm their involvement. Variations in the *CYP19A1* gene, which encodes aromatase, have been investigated, but no significant link to OHSS has been established [9, 13].
- Rare variants in *signalling pathways*, such as the integrin-linked kinase (ILK) and axonal guidance pathways, are associated with VEGF and endothelial function. These pathways are crucial in regulating vascular permeability, a key factor in OHSS [14]. The dysregulation of these pathways suggests a genetic predisposition to OHSS.
- Yan B and colleagues emphasise the significance of transcriptome profiling, which revealed multiple differentially expressed genes (DEGs) in peripheral blood, such as C3, vWF, VCAM1, and GAS6, that are linked to risk factors for OHSS. These DEGs may play a contributing role in the pathogenesis of the syndrome [15].

While genetic factors provide substantial insight into the pathogenesis of OHSS, it is crucial to acknowledge the multifactorial nature of the syndrome. Environmental factors, such as the type and dosage of gonadotropins used in assisted reproductive technologies, also play a critical role. Additionally, the interaction between genetic predispositions and these environmental factors can influence the likelihood and severity of OHSS, highlighting the complexity of its pathogenesis.

2.3 Immune Cell Involvement

While the direct role of immune cells in OHSS is not extensively documented, research into disorders related to PCOS indicates that innate immune cells, mast cells in particular, may contribute to ovarian disease processes. Moreover, circulating immune populations, especially peripheral blood mononuclear cells (PBMCs), have been found to secrete higher levels of vascular endothelial growth factor (VEGF) in patients with OHSS. These cells could potentially influence the inflammatory environment and vascular changes associated with OHSS [16]. This underscores the need for further research into their specific contributions to OHSS.

2.4 Other Molecular Mechanisms

- *Exosomal miRNAs*: Differential expression of exosomal miRNAs, such as miR-27, has been observed in OHSS patients. These miRNAs can influence oxidative stress and apoptosis in granulosa cells, potentially affecting the development and severity of OHSS [17].
- *Melatonin and receptor expression*: Elevated melatonin levels in follicular fluid and increased melatonin receptor 2 (MT2) expression in granulosa cells have been associated with OHSS. Melatonin may upregulate VEGF expression, contributing to the syndrome's pathogenesis [18].

2.5 Clinical and Demographic Factors (Table 2.2)

- *Patient demographics:* Individuals who are younger have a lower body mass index (BMI) or a known history of allergies are more likely to develop OHSS.
- *Ovarian response indicators:* Elevated serum oestradiol levels, the presence of numerous growing follicles, and the retrieval of a high number of oocytes during ART procedures are all predictive factors indicating a heightened risk of OHSS [19].

While the pathogenesis of OHSS is complex and multifactorial, the primary mechanism involves increased capillary permeability and fluid shifts, driven by hormonal and vascular factors. The identification of at-risk individuals and the implementation of preventive strategies, such as modifying stimulation protocols and using alternative ovulation triggers, are crucial for minimising both the occurrence and intensity of OHSS. Despite these insights, the complete prevention of OHSS remains challenging, highlighting the need for ongoing research and refinement of ART protocols.

Table 2.2 Risk factors of OHSS [20]

Risk factors for OHSS (Sun et al.)	
Risk factors at baseline	Risk factors during ovarian stimulation
PCOS Previous OHSS. AFC > 24. AMH level > 3.4 ng/mL. SNPs in genes involved in follicular growth (*BMP15*)	17 follicles over 10 mm at the trigger Elevated or rapidly rising estradiol at trigger (>3500 pg/mL) 15 oocytes retrieved Use of hCG for luteal support Elevated serum/follicular fluid VEGF levels regnancy (endogenous hCG)

2.6 Current Concepts in Staging

The classification or staging systems for OHSS play an important role in its diagnosis, prevention, and treatment outcomes. These systems help strategize the severity of the condition, which is essential for determining appropriate management strategies (Fig. 2.1). The current classification systems are based on clinical symptoms and laboratory findings to guide clinicians' decision-making processes. However, there are challenges and limitations associated with these systems, which can affect their effectiveness.

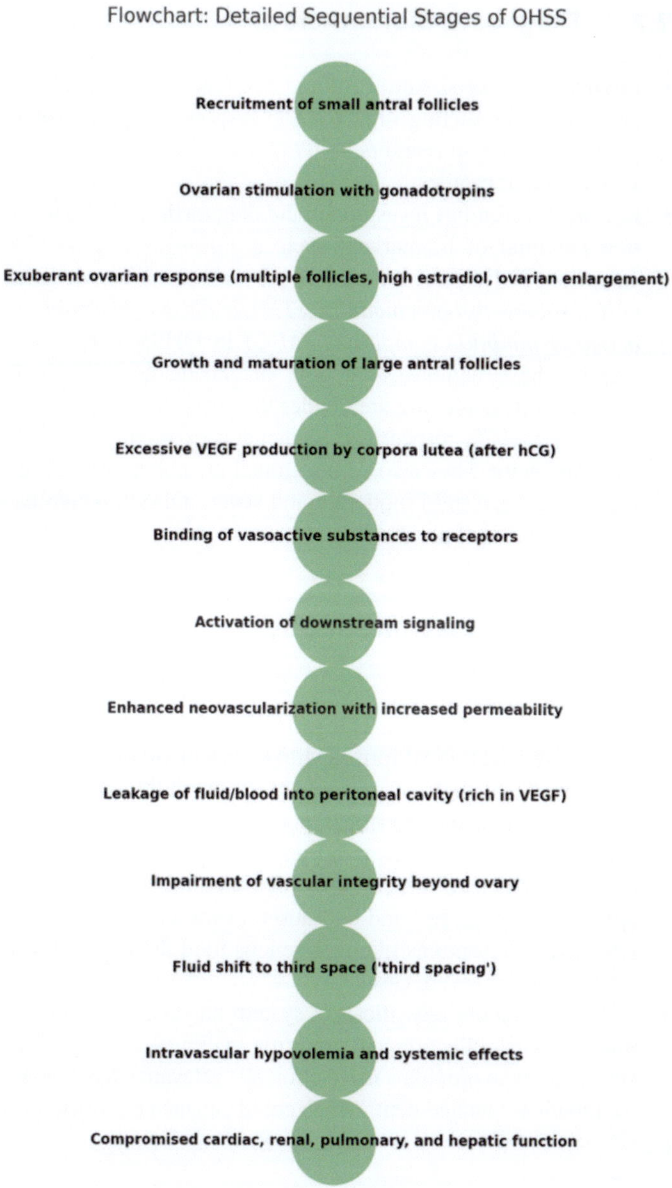

Fig. 2.1 Sequential clinical-pathophysiological stages of OHSS

2.7 Diagnostic Biomarkers and Classification

- Predictive markers: Antral follicle count and AMH levels are effective in predicting high ovarian response, a precursor to OHSS [21]. These markers help tailor COS protocols to individual patient profiles.
- Recent research has investigated the diagnostic and classification potential of biomarkers such as *thrombin-antithrombin complex (TAT), plasmin alpha2-plasmin inhibitor complex (PIC), soluble thrombomodulin (sTM), and tissue plasminogen activator-inhibitor complex (TPAI-C)* in OHSS [22]. These markers have demonstrated high diagnostic accuracy, with TAT and PIC achieving area under the curve (AUC) values of 0.991 and 0.973, respectively, indicating excellent sensitivity and specificity. They also demonstrated the potential to differentiate between mild-moderate and severe OHSS, which can predict the risk of progression to severe forms [22].

2.8 Clinical Classification Systems (Table 2.3)

- Based on symptoms and laboratory findings, traditional clinical classification systems categorise OHSS into mild, moderate, severe, and critical forms. Mild OHSS involves abdominal discomfort and slight ovarian enlargement, while severe forms of OHSS may result in critical, potentially fatal complications such as thromboembolism and renal dysfunction [23]. These classifications are crucial for determining the treatment approach, such as rest and hydration for mild cases, and more intensive interventions like intravenous fluid therapy and hospitalisation for severe cases.
- A novel inpatient classification system has been proposed to improve data collection and reporting in clinical settings. This system aims to provide a more clinically relevant classification for inpatient management, which could enhance treatment out-

Table 2.3 Current classification of OHSS [23]

	Classification of OHSS				
	Mild OHSS: characterised by bilateral multicystic ovarian enlargement		Moderate OHSS: characterised by ascites and abdominal distension	Severe OHSS: characterised by hypovolaemia, haemoconcentration, thrombosis, oliguria, pleural, and pericardial effusion	
	Grade 1	Grade 2	Grade 3	Grade 4	Grade 5
Clinical features	Abdominal distention and discomfort	Grade 1 with nausea, vomiting, and/or diarrhoea, and ovarian enlargement from 5 to 12 cm	Features of mild OHSS with ultrasonographic evidence of ascites	Presence of mild and moderate features plus: Clinical evidence of ascites (can be tense ascites) Severe abdominal pain Intractable nausea and vomiting Rapid weight gain (>1 kg in 24 h) Pleural effusion Severe dyspnoea Oliguria/anuria (<300 mL/d or < 30 mL/h) Low blood/central venous pressure Syncope Venous thrombosis	Presence of grade 4 features plus: Anuria/acute renal failure Arrhythmia Pericardial effusion Massive hydrothorax Thromboembolism Arterial thrombosis ARDS Sepsis
Laboratory features	No clinically important laboratory findings		Haemoconcentration (Hct > 41%) Leucocytosis (WBC >15,000/μL) Hypoproteinemia	Haemoconcentration (Hct > 55%) WBC >25,000/μL Serum creatinine >1.6 mg/dL Creatinine clearance <50 mL/min Hyponatremia (Na^+ < 135 mEq/L) Hyperkalemia (K^+ > 5 mEq/L) Increased liver enzymes	Worsening of biochemical findings seen with grade 4 OHSS

comes by tailoring interventions to the severity of the condition [24].
- Bayesian nonparametric models: These models cluster patients based on predictive characteristics and treatment responses, allowing for more precise treatment selection and improved outcomes in personalised medicine [25].

Clinical trial investigators in this field have proposed an alternative set of criteria for diagnosing and classifying OHSS [26].

- *Mild OHSS*: Patients exhibiting mild symptoms are categorised as "ovarian hyperresponders".
- *Moderate, severe, or critical OHSS*: Patients with moderate or more severe symptoms are classified under "OHSS", which is further subdivided into:
- *Self-limited OHSS*: Cases without any catastrophic complications.
- *OHSS with significant comorbidities*: Cases involving at least one severe complication, such as venous thromboembolism, acute respiratory distress syndrome, cerebral oedema, acute ischemia, encephalopathy, kidney injury, or liver failure.

2.9 Impact on Treatment Outcomes

- The classification of OHSS directly influences treatment strategies. For instance, severe OHSS may require hospitalisation and aggressive management to prevent life-threatening complications like thromboembolism or kidney failure.
- Preventive measures such as replacing hCG with a GnRH agonist to induce ovulation have proven effective in lowering the risk of severe OHSS. These interventions are guided by risk classification systems that assist in identifying individuals who are more likely to develop serious forms of the condition [27].
- Evidence has shown that certain stimulation protocols in ART, such as those using recombinant preparations, are associated with higher follicle counts and oocyte yields, which are critical

for assessing OHSS risk. These findings highlight the importance of selecting appropriate protocols to minimise OHSS risk [28].

2.10 Challenges and Limitations

- Despite the advancements in classification systems, there are challenges in accurately predicting the risk of severe OHSS. Established risk factors, such as polycystic ovary syndrome, do not always correlate with the severity of the condition, indicating a need for more precise predictive tools [29].
- The variability in classification criteria across different studies and clinical settings can lead to inconsistencies in diagnosis and treatment outcomes. This highlights the need for standardised classification systems that can be universally applied [5].
- While current classification systems for OHSS have significantly improved the diagnosis and management of the condition, there are still areas that require further research and development. The comparison of different risk assessment methods for OHSS reveals variations in accuracy and reliability, influenced by the methodologies and criteria used in each approach. The integration of biomarkers into these systems shows promise in enhancing diagnostic accuracy and predicting disease progression. A streamlined risk assessment index for OHSS has been suggested to better distinguish cases of moderate to severe severity. This tool is designed to improve predictive accuracy by concentrating on defined risk factors and individual patient profiles [30].
- However, the variability in classification criteria and the limitations of current risk factors underscore the need for continued efforts to refine these systems for better patient outcomes. The variability in individual responses to treatment and the complexity of integrating genomic data into clinical practice pose significant hurdles. Additionally, the lack of large-scale randomised clinical trials to validate some of the emerging

strategies highlights the need for further research to establish their efficacy and safety. Nonetheless, the ongoing development of personalised approaches holds the potential to significantly improve patient outcomes in the context of OHSS.

References

1. Bergh PA, Navot D. Ovarian hyperstimulation syndrome: a review of pathophysiology. J Assist Reprod Genet. 1992;9(5):429–38. https://doi.org/10.1007/BF01204048.
2. Soares SR, Gómez R, Simón C, García-Velasco JA, Pellicer A. Targeting the vascular endothelial growth factor system to prevent ovarian hyperstimulation syndrome. Hum Reprod Update. 2008;14(4):321–33.
3. Michele K, Elizabeth M. Pathophysiology, treatment and prevention of ovarian hyperstimulation syndrome. Curr Opin Obstet Gynecol. 2016;28(4):236–41.
4. Kumar P, Sait SF, Sharma A, Kumar M. Ovarian hyperstimulation syndrome. J Human Reprod Sci. 2011;4(2):70–5.
5. Rizk B, Aboulghar M, Smitz J, Ron-El R. The role of vascular endothelial growth factor and interleukins in the pathogenesis of severe ovarian hyperstimulation syndrome. Hum Reprod Update. 1997;3(3):255–66.
6. Gómez R, Soares SR, Busso C, Garcia-Velasco JA, Simón C, Pellicer A. Physiology and pathology of ovarian hyperstimulation syndrome. Semin Reprod Med. 2010;28(6):448–57.
7. Morris RS, Wong IL, Do YS, Hsueh WA, Lobo RA, Sauer MV, Pauslon RJ. The pathophysiology of ovarian hyperstimulation syndrome (OHSS). A proposal role of the ovarian derived prorenin to angiotensin cascade (ODPAC). Adv Exp Med Biol. 1995;377:391–8.
8. Rodien P, Beau I, Vasseur C. Ovarian hyperstimulation syndrome (OHSS) due to mutations in the follicle-stimulating hormone receptor. Ann Endocrinol. 2010;71(3):206–9.
9. Binder H, Dittrich R, Hager I, Müller A, Oeser S, Beckmann MW, Hamori M, Fasching PA, Strick R. Association of FSH receptor and CYP19A1 gene variations with sterility and ovarian hyperstimulation syndrome. Reproduction. 2008;135(1):107–16.
10. Ghaderian SM, Akbarzadeh R, Mohajerani F, Khodaii Z, Salehpour S. The implication of single-nucleotide polymorphisms in ovarian hyperstimulation syndrome. Mol Reprod Dev. 2019;86(8):964–71.
11. Wang L, Li H, Ai J, Yue J, Li Z, Zhang H, Zhao Y. Attenuated AMH signaling pathway plays an important role in the pathogenesis of ovarian hyperstimulation syndrome. Am J Transl Res. 2015;7(10):1925–38.

12. Lin H, Li Y, Xing W, Qiu Q, Wang W, Zhang Q. Genome-wide screening differential long non-coding RNAs expression profiles discloses its roles involved in OHSS development. J Assist Reprod Genet. 2018;35(8):1473–82.
13. Stouffs K, Daelemans S, Santos-Ribeiro S, Seneca S, Gheldof A, Gürbüz AS, De Vos M, Tournaye H, Blockeel C. Rare genetic variants potentially involved in ovarian hyperstimulation syndrome. J Assist Reprod Genet. 2019;36(3):491–7.
14. Borgwardt L, Olsen KW, Rossing M, Helweg-Larsen RB, Toftager M, Pinborg A, Bogstad J, Løssl K, Zedeler A, Grøndahl ML. Rare genetic variants suggest dysregulation of signalling pathways in low- and high-risk patients developing severe ovarian hyperstimulation syndrome. J Assist Reprod Genet. 2020;37(11):2883–92.
15. Yan B, Wu B, Wang Z-Q, Wei Y, Ni Y-L. Peripheral blood transcriptome analysis of patients with ovarian Hyperstimulation syndrome through high-throughput sequencing. Reprod Dev Med. 2023;7:115–21.
16. Kosaka K, Fujiwara H, Yoshioka S, Fujii S. Vascular endothelial growth factor production by circulating immune cells is elevated in ovarian hyperstimulation syndrome. Hum Reprod. 2007;22(6):1647–51.
17. Liu K, Yang W, Hu M, Xie W, Huang J, Cui M, He X, Nie X. Exosomal miR-27 negatively regulates ROS production and promotes granulosa cells apoptosis by targeting SPRY2 in OHSS. J Cell Mol Med. 2021;25(8):3976–90.
18. Li Y, Fang L, Yu Y, Shi H, Wang S, Guo Y, Sun Y. Higher melatonin in the follicle fluid and MT2 expression in the granulosa cells contribute to the OHSS occurrence. Reprod Biol Endocrinol. 2019;17:1–9.
19. Gullo G, Cucinella G, Stojanovic V, Stojkovic M, Bruno C, Streva AV, Lopez A, Perino A, Marinelli S. Ovarian Hyperstimulation syndrome (OHSS): a narrative review and legal implications. J Pers Med. 2024;14(9):915.
20. Sun B, Ma Y, Li L, Hu L, Wang F, Zhang Y, Dai S, Sun Y. Factors associated with ovarian Hyperstimulation syndrome (OHSS) severity in women with polycystic ovary syndrome undergoing IVF/ICSI. Front Endocrinol. 2020;11:615957.
21. Nastri CO, Teixeira DM, Moroni RM, Leitão VM, Martins WP. Ovarian hyperstimulation syndrome: pathophysiology, staging, prediction and prevention. Ultrasound Obstet Gynecol. 2015;45(4):377–93.
22. Li S, Qian Y, Pei Y, Wu K, Lu S. Coagulation and fibrinolysis biomarkers as potential indicators for the diagnosis and classification of ovarian Hyperstimulation syndrome. Front Med (Lausanne). 2021;8:720342.
23. Ali M, Mathur R. Ovarian hyperstimulation syndrome: a review of recent practices. Obstetr Gynaecol Reprod Med. 2023;33(1):9–13.
24. Medwin C, Rozen G, Agresta F, Nassar N, Polyakov A. The ovarian hyperstimulation that truly matters: admissions, severity and prevention strategies. Aust N Z J Obstet Gynaecol. 2023;63(4):583–7.

25. Wu D, Shi H, Yu Y, Yu T, Zhai J. Comparison of the effectiveness of various medicines in the prevention of ovarian hyperstimulation syndrome: a network meta-analysis of randomized controlled trials. Front Endocrinol (Lausanne). 2022;13:808517.
26. Humaidan P, Nelson SM, Devroey P, Coddington CC, Schwartz LB, Gordon K, Frattarelli JL, Tarlatzis BC, Fatemi HM, Lutjen P, Stegmann BJ. Ovarian hyperstimulation syndrome: review and new classification criteria for reporting in clinical trials. Hum Reprod. 2016;9:1997–2004.
27. Blumenfeld Z. The ovarian Hyperstimulation syndrome. Vitam Horm. 2018;107:423–51.
28. Stoev S, Getov I, Timeva T, Naseva EK, Lebanova H, Petkova B. Study of clinical experience with different approaches to controlled ovarian hyperstimulation: a focus on safety and efficacy. Eur J Hosp Pharm. 2021;28(1):33–7.
29. Zivi E, Simon A, Laufer N. Ovarian hyperstimulation syndrome: definition, incidence, and classification. Semin Reprod Med. 2010;28(06):441–7.
30. Cao M, Lin Q, Liu Z, Lin Y, Huang Q, Fu Y, Zhang Y, Shi H, Duan C, Liu H, Liu J. Optimized personalized management approach for moderate/severe OHSS: development and prospective validation of an OHSS risk assessment index. Hum Reprod. 2024;39(10):2320–30.

Prediction and Risk Factors of OHSS

3

Liron Seidman and Daniel S. Seidman

3.1 Introduction

Ovarian hyperstimulation syndrome (OHSS) is an iatrogenic and potentially serious complication associated with controlled ovarian stimulation (COS) in assisted reproductive technology (ART) [1, 2]. The incidence of OHSS varies significantly across ART cycles. Studies showed that mild OHSS occurs in 20–33% of ART cycles, while moderate-to-severe OHSS is observed in 3–8% of cycles [2, 3].

In recent years, significant efforts have been undertaken to reduce the incidence of this potentially avoidable complication. These efforts primarily focus on identifying women who are at higher risk for OHSS. By predicting which women are most likely to develop OHSS, it is now possible to choose safer ovarian stimulation protocols, adjust dosing, and utilize agonist triggers and new strategies such as "freeze-all." The ultimate objective of an "OHSS-free clinic" has never seemed like a realistic possibility before.

L. Seidman (✉) · D. S. Seidman
Department of Obstetrics and Gynecology, The Chaim Sheba Medical Center, Tel-Hashomer, Israel, and The Faculty of Medical & Health Sciences, Tel Aviv University, Tel Aviv, Israel

G. N. Allahbadia et al. (eds.), *Ovarian Hyperstimulation Syndrome (OHSS) Free Clinic*, https://doi.org/10.1007/978-981-95-3289-6_3

Current studies have emphasized the importance of a personalized medicine approach, demonstrating a notable reduction in the incidence of OHSS. A large national study reported a significant decline in OHSS rates between 2006 and 2015. Specifically, the overall rate of OHSS dropped from 14.3 cases per 1000 cycles in 2006 to 5.3 cases per 1000 cycles in 2015. The rate of moderate OHSS decreased from 10.5 to 4.2 cases per 1000 cycles, while the rate of severe OHSS fell from 3.83 to 1.06 cases per 1000 cycles [4].

Despite these advancements, some recent studies show that OHSS remains a concern and is far from being eradicated [3]. The financial burden associated with OHSS-related hospitalizations clearly persists. While techniques have led to a decline in OHSS admissions since 2004, this decrease has reached a plateau [3]. As a result, ongoing efforts to prevent OHSS remain necessary to further reduce the incidence of OHSS.

All clinicians recognize that OHSS can theoretically occur in any woman undergoing COS with gonadotropins. However, evidence indicates that certain women are at significantly higher risk [5]. The goal of this chapter is to identify the risk factors and personal characteristics that can assist clinicians in achieving an OHSS-free clinic.

3.1.1 Patient Characteristics

OHSS has several known risk factors, including patient characteristics that are present at baseline (Table 3.1). As these factors can be assessed before medications are administered, they are the most useful.

3.1.2 Patient Age

Patient age plays a significant role in influencing the risk of OHSS during ART treatments. In general, younger women, particularly those under the age of 35, are consistently found to be associated with a higher incidence of OHSS [6]. This increased risk is largely

Table 3.1 Patient characteristics and OHSS riske

Characteristic	Risk factor for OHSS
Age	**Higher risk in women under 35** due to higher ovarian reserve **Lower risk in women over 40** due to reduced ovarian reserve and lower response to stimulation, but **increased risk of life-threatening complications if OHSS** occurs [5, 6]
Polycystic ovary syndrome (PCOS)	High risk in women with PCOS due to elevated ovarian reserve, increased sensitivity to gonadotropins, and hormonal imbalances [7] Risk is lower in women with PCOS and metabolic syndrome
Ethnic origin	**Asian women may have** higher ovarian reserve, **increasing OHSS risk** [5] Some studies suggest higher OHSS risk in black and Hispanic women [4] Findings are inconclusive
Previous OHSS	High risk of recurrence if a patient has previously experienced OHSS [9]

due to the fact that younger women tend to have a higher ovarian reserve, meaning they have more follicles capable of responding to stimulation by gonadotropins. A higher ovarian reserve often leads to a stronger response to the fertility medications used in COS, which increases the likelihood of OHSS.

Younger women often have elevated levels of anti-Müllerian hormone (AMH), an indicator of ovarian reserve, which can make their ovaries more responsive to stimulation. This heightened sensitivity results in the production of many follicles and increased estradiol levels, both of which are risk factors for OHSS.

In contrast, older women, particularly those over 40, are generally at a lower risk of OHSS. This is because ovarian reserve naturally declines with age, leading to a reduced number of follicles and a less vigorous response to stimulation. However, age-related factors such as reduced ovarian function can necessitate higher doses of gonadotropins to achieve sufficient follicular development, further lowering the risk of overstimulation. Thus, although young age was linked with an increased risk of OHSS, among individuals hospitalized with severe OHSS, patients older than 40 years were at increased risk for life-threatening complications [5].

3.2 Polycystic Ovarian Syndrome

Polycystic ovary syndrome (PCOS) significantly increases the risk of OHSS during fertility treatments, particularly in ART. In a study of 2699 women with PCOS who underwent ART, almost one in four (24.8%) developed OHSS in response to COH [7]. This heightened risk stems from the hormonal and ovarian characteristics associated with PCOS, which predispose women to an exaggerated response to the gonadotropins used in COS.

Additionally, women with PCOS often experience irregular ovulatory cycles and hormonal imbalances, including elevated luteinizing hormone (LH) levels and insulin resistance. These factors can complicate the body's response to fertility medications, making it more difficult to predict the ovarian response and increasing the likelihood of overstimulation.

Women with PCOS typically have a higher ovarian reserve, characterized by a large number of small antral follicles. These follicles are highly sensitive to the stimulation provided by gonadotropins, often leading to excessive follicular development. When many follicles mature simultaneously, there is an increase in estradiol levels, which contribute to the fluid shift from the blood vessels to body cavities—a key mechanism in the development of OHSS. It was found that a high antral follicle count (AFC) was a strong marker of OHSS, while basal serum E2 was the best predictor of OHSS severity in women with PCOS undergoing IVF treatment [7].

Among women with PCOS, those with metabolic syndrome appear to be at a lower OHSS risk than those without. In some studies, body mass index (BMI) was shown to be negatively associated with OHSS risk, while in others, no relationship was found between BMI and OHSS risk [5]. Body mass index and lean body weight, however, are unreliable indicators of OHSS [8].

In summary, the high ovarian reserve, hormonal imbalances, and heightened sensitivity to stimulation in women with PCOS make them more susceptible to OHSS during fertility treatments. Special care in monitoring and selecting the right stimulation protocols is essential for reducing the risk in these patients.

3.3 Ethnic Origin

The association between ethnic origin and the risk for OHSS is not fully understood, though some research suggests that certain ethnic groups may have varying levels of risk due to genetic, physiological, and environmental factors. For example, women of different ethnic backgrounds may have differences in ovarian reserve, such as higher AFC or AMH levels. These differences can influence their response to gonadotropins during COS. Some studies have suggested that women of Asian origin may have higher ovarian reserves, potentially increasing their risk for OHSS. Additionally, genetic variants related to ovarian function and hormone receptors, such as FSH receptor gene variants, may be more common in certain ethnic groups, potentially influencing the risk of OHSS.

While there is some data suggesting differences in OHSS rates among ethnic groups, the findings have been inconclusive, and studies exploring the relationship between ethnicity and OHSS risk are limited. It was reported that the risk of developing OHSS for black women was greater than for white women, while for Hispanic women, the risk was lower [5]. Another study found that non-Hispanic black and Hispanic women were at an increased risk of OHSS compared with non-Hispanic white women [4]. Most large-scale studies, however, have not consistently included detailed analyses across various ethnic groups, making it difficult to draw definitive conclusions about the role of ethnicity in OHSS risk. Further research is needed to better understand how ethnicity may influence OHSS susceptibility.

Cultural and environmental factors could also play a role in OHSS risk. Access to fertility care and treatment approaches may differ across ethnic groups, influenced by cultural, socioeconomic, or regional factors. These differences may impact the frequency or severity of OHSS, as treatment protocols and patient behaviors can vary based on these norms. Additionally, body mass index (BMI), which is a known risk factor for OHSS, varies across ethnic groups and could indirectly affect OHSS risk.

In summary, while ethnic origin may contribute to OHSS risk due to a combination of genetic, physiological, and environmental factors, there is insufficient consistent evidence to draw definitive conclusions. It seems that ethnicity alone has a limited value when assessing a patient's likelihood of developing OHSS.

3.4 Previous OHSS

A previous occurrence of OHSS substantially increases the risk of it happening again in future fertility treatments [2]. This is largely due to the persistence of the underlying factors that contributed to the initial episode. For example, women with high ovarian reserve, indicated by elevated AMH levels or a large antral follicle count, are more likely to have an excessive ovarian response during COS. Additionally, conditions such as PCOS are closely associated with an exaggerated response to ovarian stimulation, making women with PCOS more prone to developing OHSS again [9].

Women who have previously experienced OHSS may also demonstrate heightened sensitivity to gonadotropins used in ART. This sensitivity can result in the ovaries over-responding to stimulation, even when adjustments are made to lower the dosage or alter the type of hormonal trigger used. While strategies such as using a GnRH agonist trigger instead of human chorionic gonadotropin (hCG) or opting for a "freeze-all" approach (freezing embryos for later transfer) may reduce the risk, the predisposition to OHSS does not completely disappear after an initial episode.

The risk of recurrent OHSS poses significant clinical challenges, so clinicians must exercise caution in subsequent cycles, often adopting more conservative stimulation protocols and carefully monitoring estradiol levels and follicle development to mitigate the risk of recurrence. Despite these preventive measures, the increased likelihood of OHSS remains a concern, emphasizing the need for close monitoring and personalized treatment approaches for women who have previously experienced the condition.

3.5 Ovarian Reserve Markers

While demographics can provide initial insights for risk assessment, ovarian reserve markers such as AMH and AFC have consistently shown greater predictive accuracy for assessing the risk of OHSS during fertility treatments (Table 3.2). These markers provide insight into a woman's ovarian capacity, particularly her response to gonadotropin stimulation, which directly impacts her risk for developing OHSS.

Anti-Müllerian hormone levels and AFC were extensively studied as predictors of ovarian stimulation response, with various thresholds indicating a heightened risk of developing OHSS [1]. AMH levels cutoff of 24 pmol/L was found to be a good predictor of OHSS in a prospective study of women undergoing IVF stimulation, with a sensitivity of 90.5% and a specificity of 81.3% [10]. Antral follicle count is another marker of ovarian reserve closely linked to AMH levels and exhibits a similar association with

Table 3.2 Ovarian reserve markers and OHSS risk

Ovarian reserve marker	Risk factor for OHSS
Anti-Müllerian hormone (AMH)	Higher AMH levels are strongly associated with increased OHSS risk AMH levels >22.5–35 pmol/L has a strong predictive value in GnRH antagonist cycles [11]
Antral follicle count (AFC)	AFC > 20–24 is a strong predictor in GnRH antagonist cycles [5, 10]
Estradiol levels (E2)	Peak estradiol levels were not shown to be predictive of OHSS Day 3 estradiol >126 ng/mL and significant increases (more than 19×) from days 3–10 are associated with higher OHSS risk [12]
Number of oocytes retrieved	More than 13.5 oocytes retrieved is a strong predictor of OHSS risk [11]

OHSS risk. Based on a prospective study of 1012 women who had their first IVF cycle, women with an AFC >24 were at an 8.6% risk of OHSS as compared to a 2.2% risk for those who had an AFC <24 [5].

It was also demonstrated that high AMH (>35 pmol/L) and/or AFC (of 20 or more) are better predictors for OHSS compared with ovarian response parameters in current GnRH antagonist cycles [11]. Peak levels of estradiol were shown to have no predictive value according to another retrospective cohort study [11]. It was concluded that the optimal thresholds for predicting OHSS were 22.5 pmol/L for AMH (sensitivity 87.5%, specificity 60.6%), 19.5 for AFC (sensitivity 70.8%, specificity 67%), and 9.5 for the number if oocytes retrieved (sensitivity 83.5%, specificity 62.7%) [11].

A retrospective review, aimed to assess IVF parameters associated with OHSS, found OHSS patients had significantly higher day 3 E2 levels (>126 ng/mL), as well as a greater increase in serum E2 levels from day 3 to day 10. This was especially notable if the E2 concentration increased by more than 19 times [12]. Another parameter that was found to be associated with a greater risk of OHSS was a high number of ova collected (>13.5). It was found to be the best predictor with a high accuracy and specificity of 76.5% and 73.5%, respectively [11].

Moreover, the authors suggest that preventive measures should be based on ovarian reserve parameters rather than ovarian response to COH. This is because patients with high ovarian reserves are at risk for OHSS, even if their ovarian response is not excessively high [11].

In summary, higher levels of AMH and AFC are strongly associated with increased OHSS risk. These markers are valuable tools for predicting OHSS risk and guiding individualized treatment strategies to minimize the occurrence of OHSS in patients undergoing fertility treatments.

3.6 Genetic Predictors

Genetic predictors of OHSS are gaining attention as a means to identify women who are at increased risk of developing this condition during fertility treatments. One of the most extensively studied genetic markers is the FSH receptor (*FSHR*) gene, specifically the N680S polymorphism. This variation affects the sensitivity of ovarian follicles to FSH, which can lead to an exaggerated ovarian response during controlled COS. Studies have shown that women with the N680S variant are at a significantly higher risk of developing OHSS, with an odds ratio (OR) of around 1.7, meaning they are 70% more likely to experience OHSS compared to those without this genetic variant. In other studies, the FSHR Asn680Ser polymorphism predicted OHSS severity, but not which patients would develop it [13].

In addition to the FSH receptor, genes involved in the vascular endothelial growth factor (VEGF) pathway, such as FLT4, have been linked to OHSS risk. VEGF plays a critical role in blood vessel formation and permeability, processes that are central to the pathophysiology of OHSS. Variants in the *FLT4* gene, which encodes a tyrosine kinase receptor for VEGF, have been identified in women with OHSS. A case series of four individuals with OHSS, who underwent whole exome sequencing, identified a novel association between variants in the *FLT4* gene and the development of OHSS [5, 14]. These genetic changes are thought to contribute to abnormal vascular permeability, increasing the likelihood of fluid accumulation and other OHSS-related complications.

Other genetic factors being explored include variations in genes related to LH and other gonadotropins, which may further affect ovarian response during stimulation. Although these associations are still under investigation, they represent another potential genetic component influencing OHSS susceptibility. Similarly, polymorphisms in the *CYP19A1* gene, which is involved in estrogen synthesis, could also impact ovarian response and increase OHSS risk by affecting estrogen metabolism during fertility treatments.

Overall, the identification of genetic markers such as the N680S polymorphism in the FSH receptor gene and variants in VEGF-related pathways provides valuable insights into individual susceptibility to OHSS. This growing understanding of genetic predisposition allows for more personalized fertility treatments, where protocols can be adjusted to minimize the risk of OHSS based on a patient's genetic profile.

While these genetic predictors show promise, the results of genetic variant studies have been inconsistent, with some failing to replicate the findings. Therefore, genetic markers are not yet routinely used in clinical practice. Further large-scale studies are needed to validate the predictive value and to determine their utility as genetic predictors of OHSS. In conclusion, while genetic factors may play a role in OHSS susceptibility, their predictive value remains limited compared to other clinical markers [15].

3.7 Personalized Stimulation-Related Factors

Identifying individuals at increased risk of OHSS is essential for implementing proactive strategies to reduce or prevent its occurrence. Furthermore, early identification enables targeted counseling of patients in advance, informing them about their specific risks.

Although identifying individuals at increased risk of OHSS before treatment is ideal, stimulation-related factors can also help identify those at risk. As noted above, there is a positive correlation between the number of oocytes retrieved and the likelihood of developing OHSS; specifically, when 15–18 or more oocytes are retrieved, the risk significantly increases [1, 5]. In line with the number of retrieved oocytes, an elevated total count of large follicles consistently predicts OHSS risk. A total follicle count exceeding 17 was found to be an independent risk factor for OHSS [5]. Similarly, heightened serum estradiol levels at the time of ovulatory induction have been linked to OHSS risk. While the definition of elevated estradiol varies across studies, it typically falls within the 3500–5000 pg/mL range [5].

Lastly, there are ovarian stimulation-related factors that cause OHSS. The key trigger for OHSS is the administration of human chorionic gonadotropin (hCG) to induce final follicular maturation and ovulation. Therefore, OHSS can be reduced or prevented by the use of GnRH antagonist protocols with GnRH agonists used as a trigger before oocyte aspiration [2]. However, in GnRH agonist cycles, early OHSS can only be fully prevented by canceling the cycle and withholding hCG. The financial cost of treatment and the emotional impact on the patient have resulted in a major decrease in the use of GnRH agonist cycles.

Individualization of gonadotropin protocols can reduce the risk of OHSS in several keyways. First, personalized dosing based on patient characteristics. The dosing is tailored to each patient's specific factors, like AMH levels, antral follicle count, body weight, and age. This allows for more precise stimulation matched to the individual's expected ovarian response. Second, individualized protocols often result in lower total doses of gonadotropins used, especially in potential high responders, reducing the risk of overstimulation. Third, optimizing ovarian response. The goal is to achieve an adequate number of oocytes (around 7–10) while avoiding excessive stimulation. This "goldilocks" approach balances efficacy and safety. Studies have shown decreased rates of excessive ovarian response (>15 or > 20 oocytes retrieved) with individualized protocols compared to standard dosing. Multiple studies have demonstrated a significant reduction (approximately 25–50%) in early OHSS risk with individualized approaches. Such protocols can reduce the need for additional OHSS preventive measures like cycle cancellation or coasting.

Once the personalized dose is determined, it often remains fixed throughout stimulation, avoiding sudden changes that could increase OHSS risk. Younger patients with high AMH and lower body weight may particularly benefit from this tailored approach.

By providing a more controlled and patient-specific approach to ovarian stimulation, individualized gonadotropin protocols aim to improve overall treatment safety while maintaining efficacy. This approach is particularly beneficial for patients at higher risk of OHSS, helping to mitigate that risk from the start of treatment.

3.8 Algorithms and Predictive Models

Algorithms and predictive models for OHSS are becoming increasingly important tools in reproductive medicine, particularly in the context of personalized fertility treatment. These models aim to predict which patients are at higher risk of developing OHSS based on various clinical and biological factors, allowing clinicians to adjust stimulation protocols and reduce the likelihood of this potentially dangerous complication.

3.9 Single-Predictor Models

Specific algorithms were developed to estimate OHSS risk by focusing on the critical days of ovarian stimulation, such as the day of hCG trigger. For example, the ratio of estradiol to the number of follicles, or the rapid rise in estradiol levels during stimulation, is often incorporated into predictive tools. The best single predictor of severe OHSS was found to be the total number of follicles ≥10 mm on the day of hCG administration. A cutoff of ≥15 follicles ≥10 mm had high sensitivity (89.5%) and specificity (64.2%) for predicting severe OHSS [16].

3.10 Multivariable Prediction Models

Multiphase prediction models were developed to identify moderate and severe OHSS based on a retrospective cohort database of 17,445 women. These models use predefined thresholds for estradiol levels and follicle counts to predict the likelihood of OHSS, prompting clinicians to adjust the dose or switch to a GnRH agonist trigger to minimize risk. The models evaluated the baseline clinical characteristics, COS-related characteristics, and embryo information. The final model had a C-statistic of 0.814, indicating good discriminative ability. The multiphase prediction models were implemented as a user-friendly smartphone-based app for the personalized management of women at risk of OHSS. It can be used for clinical decision support and self-management of patients [17].

3.11 Decision-Making Algorithms

A retrospective study developed a decision-making tool for doctors that predicts severe OHSS early in the IVF/ICSI process. The study describes a novel decision-making algorithm based on ascites, hematocrit, white blood cell, and maximal ovarian diameter (MOD) measurements on day 3 after oocyte retrieval. The model designed to predict the probability of severe OHSS development on day 5 had an AUC of 0.93 with a sensitivity of 88.5% and a specificity of 84.2%. This algorithm can assist clinicians in making decisions on whether to proceed or cancel embryo transfers in high-risk patients triggered with hCG [18].

3.12 Personalized Dosing Algorithms

By utilizing a personalized approach, the appropriate treatment can be selected and adapted for each patient. Risks can be minimized when standardized treatment is assigned to patient groups (for example, setting doses by weight category), thereby avoiding possible complications, including OHSS [17, 19].

Algorithms have been developed to personalize dosing based on patient characteristics. The algorithm determines the optimal dose for each patient based on their serum AMH levels and body weight. This allows for more precise dosing tailored to the individual's expected ovarian response. Moreover, by individualizing the dose, the algorithm aims to achieve an adequate number of oocytes (around 7–10) while minimizing the risk of hypo- or hyperresponse/excessive ovarian stimulation, especially in potential high responders.

Multiple studies have demonstrated an approximately 25–50% relative reduction in the early OHSS risk with individualized gonadotropins compared to conventional dosing approaches. The algorithm's carefully individualized dosing regimen has been shown to reduce the need for additional preventive interventions for OHSS, such as cycle cancellation or coasting.

A prospective, uncontrolled, international, 18-center study was performed to optimize the initial FSH dose in controlled ovarian hyperstimulation and enhance IVF protocols by predicting the effectiveness of each day of COS monitoring. In the CONSORT dosing algorithm, starting gonadotropin doses are individualized based on basal FSH, body mass index, age, and the number of antral follicles in the patient. The use of the CONSORT algorithm achieved an adequate oocyte yield and good pregnancy rates in this preliminary study. The development and adjustment of these algorithms focus on predictive accuracy and prioritize patient safety and treatment effectiveness, and thereby could lead to a reduction in cancellations [20].

While these algorithms show promise, it's important to note that predicting OHSS remains challenging, especially for late-onset cases. The most reliable predictions tend to come later in the stimulation cycle when the ovarian response is known. Clinicians should use these tools with clinical judgment and other established risk factors.

3.13 Artificial Intelligence (AI)

With the rise of artificial intelligence (AI) and machine learning, newer predictive models have been developed to refine the assessment of OHSS risk. These models can analyze large datasets, including patient demographics, hormonal profiles, stimulation parameters, and genetic factors, to predict OHSS with greater accuracy. Machine learning algorithms can identify complex patterns and interactions among multiple risk factors that might be overlooked by traditional statistical models. Some AI-driven models even provide real-time risk assessments during ovarian stimulation cycles, allowing for more responsive adjustments to treatment protocols.

The integration of AI and deep learning offers the potential for developing more accurate predictive models for gonadotropin starting doses in the future. In recent years, deep learning, a key branch of AI, has been widely applied in the medical field, particularly in automated diagnoses based on clinical imaging and large-scale screening [21].

While research into predictive AI algorithms for OHSS is still in its early stages, primarily focused on retrospective analyses, further validation and prospective studies are required before these models can be broadly adopted in clinical practice. Although AI and machine learning hold promise for predicting OHSS risk, they are not yet routinely used in OHSS prevention. Nonetheless, the development of these models marks an important step toward more personalized and effective prevention strategies in assisted reproductive treatments [22].

In conclusion, algorithms and predictive models for OHSS have evolved from basic clinical risk assessment tools to complex AI-based systems that integrate genetic, hormonal, and clinical data. These models help clinicians identify high-risk patients early in the treatment cycle, enabling personalized treatment plans that minimize the risk of OHSS.

References

1. Sopa N, Larsen CE, Hvidman WH, Andersen NA. An AMH-based FSH dosing algorithm for OHSS risk reduction in first cycle antagonist protocol for IVF/ICSI. Eur J Obstet Gynecol Reprod Biol. 2019;237:42–7.
2. Braam CS, Bruin DPJ, Mol JWB, Wely VM. The perspective of women with an increased risk of OHSS regarding the safety and burden of IVF: a discrete choice experiment. Human Reprod Open. 2020;2020
3. Rotshenker-Olshinka K, Badeghiesh A, Volodarsky-Perel A, Steiner N, Suarthana E, Dahan HM. Trends in ovarian hyperstimulation syndrome hospitalization rates in the USA: an ongoing concern. Reprod Biomed Online. 2020;41:357–60.
4. Schirmer AD, Kulkarni DA, Zhang Y, Kawwass FJ, Boulet LS, Kissin MD. Ovarian hyperstimulation syndrome after assisted reproductive technologies: trends, predictors, and pregnancy outcomes. Fertil Steril. 2020;114:567–78.
5. Medicine PCotASfR. Prevention of moderate and severe ovarian hyperstimulation syndrome: a guideline. Fertil Steril. 2024;121:230–45.
6. Whelan GJ, Vlahos FN. The ovarian hyperstimulation syndrome. Fertil Steril. 2000;73:883–96.

7. Sun B, Ma Y, Li L, et al. Factors associated with ovarian hyperstimulation syndrome (OHSS) severity in women with polycystic ovary syndrome undergoing IVF/ICSI. Front Endocrinol. 2021;11
8. Lewis GC, Warnes MG, Wang X, Matthews DC. Failure of body mass index or body weight to influence markedly the response to ovarian hyperstimulation in normal cycling women. Fertil Steril. 1990;53:1097–9.
9. Humaidan P, Nelson SM, Devroey P, et al. Ovarian hyperstimulation syndrome: review and new classification criteria for reporting in clinical trials. Hum Reprod. 2016;31:1997–2004.
10. Lee T-H, Liu C-H, Huang C-C, et al. Serum anti-mullerian hormone and estradiol levels as predictors of ovarian hyperstimulation syndrome in assisted reproduction technology cycles. Hum Reprod. 2007;23:160–7.
11. Sood A, Goel A, Boda S, Mathur R. Prediction of significant OHSS by ovarian reserve and ovarian response – implications for elective freeze-all strategy. Hum Fertil. 2022;25:390–6.
12. Madrazo I, Vélez FM, Hidalgo JJ, et al. Prediction of severe ovarian hyperstimulation syndrome in women undergoing in vitro fertilization using estradiol levels, collected ova, and number of follicles. J Int Med Res. 2020;48:030006052094555.
13. Daelemans C, Smits G, Maertelaer DV, et al. Prediction of severity of symptoms in iatrogenic ovarian hyperstimulation syndrome by follicle-stimulating hormone receptor Ser_{680}Asn polymorphism. J Clin Endocrinol Metabol. 2004;89:6310–5.
14. Stouffs K, Daelemans S, Santos-Ribeiro S, et al. Rare genetic variants potentially involved in ovarian hyperstimulation syndrome. J Assist Reprod Genet. 2019;36:491–7.
15. Altmäe S, Hovatta O, Stavreus-Evers A, Salumets A. Genetic predictors of controlled ovarian hyperstimulation: where do we stand today? Hum Reprod Update. 2011;17:813–28.
16. Tarlatzi BT, Venetis AC, Devreker F, Englert Y, Delbaere A. What is the best predictor of severe ovarian hyperstimulation syndrome in IVF? A cohort study. J Assist Reprod Genet. 2017;34:1341–51.
17. Cao M, Liu Z, Lin Y, et al. A personalized management approach of OHSS: development of a multiphase prediction model and smartphone-based app. Front Endocrinol. 2022;13:91225.
18. Lainas G, Lainas T, Sfontouris I, et al. A decision-making algorithm for performing or cancelling embryo transfer in patients at high risk for ovarian hyperstimulation syndrome after triggering final oocyte maturation with hCG. Human Reprod Open. 2020;2020
19. Fiedler K, Ezcurra D. Predicting and preventing ovarian hyperstimulation syndrome (OHSS): the need for individualized not standardized treatment. Reprod Biol Endocrinol. 2012;10:32.

20. Olivennes F, Howles C, Borini A, et al. Individualizing FSH dose for assisted reproduction using a novel algorithm: the CONSORT study. Reprod Biomed Online. 2009;18:195–204.
21. Guo X, Zhan H, Zhang X, et al. Predictive models for starting dose of gonadotropin in controlled ovarian hyperstimulation: review and progress update. Hum Fertil. 2023;26:1609–16.
22. Ziaee A, Khosravi H, Sadeghi T, Ahmed I, Mahmoudinia M. Prediction of complicated ovarian hyperstimulation syndrome in assisted reproductive treatment through artificial intelligence, 2024, medRxiv preprint https://doi.org/10.1101/2024.04.17.24305980.

Primary and Secondary OHSS

4

Akanksha Allahbadia Gupta,
Swati Gautam Allahbadia,
and Gautam Nand Allahbadia

4.1 Introduction

OHSS is an iatrogenic complication that can cause significant morbidity in its severe or critical form. The incidence of clinically severe OHSS is approximately 2–3%, with mild forms observed in about 20–30% of IVF cases. It is classified as early or primary when occurring within 8 days of gonadotropin stimulation, and late or secondary when presenting after 9 days—mainly relating to endogenous hCG during pregnancy. Rare cases of spontaneous OHSS have been documented. These, along with early-onset followed by late-onset OHSS, are the most severe [1].

A. A. Gupta (✉)
Sumitra Hospital, Noida, Uttar Pradesh, India

S. G. Allahbadia
Rotunda – The Center for Human Reproduction,
Wadala (West), Mumbai, Maharashtra, India

G. N. Allahbadia
Allahbadia Fertility Clinic, Dubai, United Arab Emirates

G. N. Allahbadia et al. (eds.), *Ovarian Hyperstimulation Syndrome (OHSS) Free Clinic*, https://doi.org/10.1007/978-981-95-3289-6_4

4.2 Pathophysiology of Ovarian Hyperstimulation Syndrome (OHSS)

Ovarian hyperstimulation occurs due to an exaggerated ovarian response to gonadotropins. While the exact pathophysiology remains unclear, the key mechanism appears to be increased capillary permeability, which causes fluid to shift from the intravascular compartment to the third space [2]. The ovaries enlarge in size, thus increasing the risk of torsion or hemorrhage. Accumulation of fluid in the third space can lead to peripheral edema, ascites, pleural effusion, or pericardial effusion. As a result, intravascular volume depletion occurs, leading to hypotension and oliguria and raising the risk of thromboembolic events. In severe cases, renal or respiratory failure and even death may occur [3].

Although the pathogenesis is not fully understood, vascular endothelial growth factor (VEGF) is thought to play a central role [3]. VEGF expression is stimulated by hCG and is found to be elevated in OHSS cases. Its strong influence on vascular permeability has been well established, and inhibition of VEGF action in affected individuals has been shown to reduce or prevent OHSS symptoms [4].

Previously, hCG was considered essential for OHSS development, but recent case studies have shown that it can occur in its absence. Other contributing factors under investigation include impaired anti-Müllerian hormone (AMH) signaling and immune cell involvement—specifically $CD11c^{+}HLA\text{-}DR^{+}$ dendritic cells and associated interleukins [5].

Early-onset OHSS is typically related to an immediate ovarian over-response to gonadotropin stimulation, often when ovulation is triggered with hCG. In contrast, late-onset OHSS is associated with hCG produced endogenously by the trophoblast after embryo implantation [6].

A study involving 4250 women undergoing IVF/ICSI classified OHSS cases by timing of onset. Endogenous hCG appears in the maternal serum around 8–10 days after administration of exogenous hCG, which simulates the natural LH surge. Thus, early-onset OHSS occurs between days 1 and 10 following hCG administration, whereas late-onset OHSS presents between days 13 and 38. The same study suggested that those with early-onset OHSS who become pregnant may face a poorer prognosis than those who experience late-onset OHSS [7].

4.2.1 Risk Factors for OHSS

Various factors increase the likelihood of developing OHSS. These include being under 30 years of age [8], having a low body mass index, polycystic ovary syndrome (PCOS), or a high baseline antral follicle count (AFC) [9]. Rapidly rising or high estradiol levels during ovarian stimulation are also risk factors [2, 10]. A personal history of excessive response to gonadotropins, including prior OHSS, also contributes [11]. The presence of many small follicles (8–12 mm) during stimulation [12], use of hCG instead of progesterone for luteal support [13], a high number of oocytes retrieved [14], early pregnancy [15], and elevated basal AMH levels [16] are additional risk factors. Ethnicity may also play a role, with African-American women having a higher reported risk compared to Hispanic or Caucasian women [17].

Evidence strongly supports that markers of high ovarian responsiveness increase OHSS risk. Key factors include younger age and a PCOS diagnosis, as well as elevated ovarian reserve markers like AFC greater than 24 and AMH above 3.4 ng/mL [17].

Stimulation-related risks include:

- More than 17–19 mature follicles at the time of trigger.
- Estradiol levels above 3500–5000 pg/mL at trigger.
- Retrieval of more than 15–18 oocytes.

Random-start stimulation protocols are helpful in fertility settings where no fresh transfer is intended. In these cases, early detection of unintended pregnancy via serial hCG measurements is recommended. Delaying stimulation until pregnancy is ruled out is especially important for fertile populations like oocyte donors to avoid severe OHSS [16].

The severity of OHSS differs between singleton and multiple pregnancies. Evidence suggests that more gestational sacs are associated with greater OHSS severity, regardless of whether onset is early or late [7].

4.2.2 Clinical Discussion

Ovarian hyperstimulation syndrome (OHSS) is classified into mild, moderate, severe, or critical categories based on symptom grading, severity, and laboratory findings. It is also categorized by onset timing—early or late onset OHSS [16]. Early-onset OHSS typically arises 4–7 days following the administration of an ovulatory hCG dose during controlled ovarian stimulation. These symptoms generally resolve with the onset of menstruation. In contrast, late-onset OHSS usually appears 9 or more days after the hCG trigger due to rising endogenous hCG levels during early pregnancy. This OHSS form is much more severe and has a more prolonged course.

Severe OHSS is a medical emergency that can result in complications such as pleural effusion, acute kidney injury, and venous thromboembolism [17]. It often involves rapid intraperitoneal fluid accumulation—ranging from 1.5 to 17 L—which may cause organ dysfunction including respiratory compromise and decreased urine output. In a study done on 20 patients who developed moderate to severe OHSS, intra-abdominal pressure (IAP) was elevated into pathological ranges. These findings suggest that OHSS can function as a compartment syndrome and, in advanced presentations, meet criteria for abdominal compartment syndrome. Consequently, managing severe OHSS should include pressure reduction via paracentesis to prevent complications and worsening of the condition [17].

OHSS prevention is targeted based on its stage and is divided into a primary and a secondary strategy [8]. Primary prevention aims to tailor stimulation protocols based on individual risk factors.

Women at elevated risk—such as those with PCOS, a personal or family history of OHSS or thromboembolism, thrombophilia, or antiphospholipid antibodies—should be identified early. In such cases, treatment should begin with the minimum effective dose of gonadotropins, coupled with close monitoring via serial vaginal ultrasounds and/or serum estradiol assessments.

One of the cornerstone primary prevention methods involves using a GnRH antagonist protocol. For secondary prevention—meant for patients who show an excessive response during stimulation—the most effective recent approach is the use of a GnRH agonist (GnRHa) trigger for final oocyte maturation. This method ensures adequate oocyte maturation while significantly reducing or even eliminating the risk of OHSS.

A newer approach involves the use of kisspeptin to induce oocyte maturation in high-risk patients. Although promising, additional evidence is required to fully assess its efficacy and safety profile [18]. Kisspeptins primarily act on the hypothalamus by stimulating Kiss1 neurons, which regulate the pulsatile release of GnRH and thereby influence gonadotropin release and ovarian function. Other potential action sites along the hypothalamic-pituitary-ovarian (HPO) axis, such as the pituitary gland and ovary, have also been proposed; however, the physiologic significance of these extrahypothalamic actions remains uncertain [19].

It is essential to counsel women on the natural progression of OHSS, particularly regarding the extended duration of symptoms if pregnancy occurs. While most hospitalizations are brief, in some cases they can extend up to 4 weeks [20].

Spontaneous OHSS is extremely rare and is almost exclusively observed during pregnancy. It has been reported in association with multiple gestations [21] or hydatidiform moles, both of which are known to produce unusually high levels of hCG [22]. Additionally, cases linked to hypothyroidism suggest that elevated thyroid-stimulating hormone (TSH) levels may also stimulate ovarian activity [23]. Some patients experience recurrent spontaneous OHSS across two to six successive pregnancies [24]. Unlike iatrogenic OHSS, which typically emerges between 3 and 5 weeks of amenorrhea, spontaneous forms usually develop between 8 and 14 weeks.

4.2.3 Clinical Outcomes

A 15-year retrospective study conducted between 2000 and 2015 evaluated the clinical outcomes associated with OHSS in both fresh and frozen embryo transfer cycles [25]. Among singleton IVF pregnancies, OHSS was associated with an increased risk of low birth weight (adjusted relative risk [aRR] 1.29) and preterm delivery (aRR 1.32). In twin pregnancies, the syndrome was linked to heightened risks of second-trimester pregnancy loss (aRR 1.81), low birth weight (aRR 1.06), and preterm birth (aRR 1.16). Overall, patients affected by OHSS demonstrated elevated risks of adverse perinatal outcomes such as preterm delivery and fetal growth restriction. These findings underscore the importance of implementing preventative strategies in clinical practice to reduce the incidence of OHSS [25].

4.2.4 Recent Advances

The ‘freeze all strategy,’ also known as ‘freeze-only,’ refers to IVF cycles where all embryos are cryopreserved for future transfer in unstimulated cycles. This method offers potential benefits such as improved implantation outcomes and the near-elimination of OHSS risk [26]. With advancing vitrification techniques, this approach is especially useful in individuals with PCOS or high ovarian response, where numerous oocytes are retrieved. The strategy prevents further ovarian stimulation by gestational hCG and is particularly protective in cases with high oocyte yield and multiple gestational sacs [27].

Intravenous calcium supplementation has also been explored for OHSS prevention. It has been shown to effectively reduce the incidence of moderate or severe OHSS without adversely affecting pregnancy rates. This supports a proposed pathophysiological model where membrane depolarization contributes to OHSS development, and calcium serves to stabilize the membrane, mitigating symptoms [28].

Two randomized trials have investigated the use of aspirin or OHSS prevention [29, 30]. Evidence suggests a beneficial effect, as one study showed reduced OHSS rates with aspirin alone compared to no treatment, while another showed benefits with a combination of acetylsalicylic acid and corticosteroids [31].

A recent meta-analysis of 12 studies involving 1516 participants indicated that while metformin use did not significantly affect pregnancy, live birth, or miscarriage rates, it was associated with a markedly reduced OHSS risk (RR 0.44; 95% CI 0.26–0.77). This provides strong support for metformin as an OHSS-reducing agent, particularly in PCOS patients [32].

In the context of establishing OHSS-free clinics, additional strategies include the use of GnRH antagonists in the luteal phase as a tertiary-level intervention for established severe OHSS. This is used alongside primary prevention (antagonist protocols) and secondary prevention (GnRH agonist trigger with or without low-dose hCG) [16]. Evidence also suggests that reproductive outcomes may be optimized when a low dose of hCG is coadministered with the GnRH agonist trigger [33].

Administration of cabergoline, a dopamine agonist, has been shown to reduce OHSS incidence without impacting pregnancy rates. A review of seven studies involving 858 patients demonstrated a significant reduction in OHSS risk (RR 0.38, 95% CI 0.29–0.51), while maintaining comparable pregnancy outcomes (RR 1.02, 95% CI 0.78–1.34). The proposed mechanism involves selective inhibition of VEGF-induced vascular permeability, possibly mediated by reduced VEGFR-2 phosphorylation, although the exact process remains under investigation [34].

A randomized, assessor-blind trial involving 347 Japanese women undergoing their first IVF/ICSI cycle compared follitropin beta with individualized follitropin delta dosing. The delta protocol, based on anti-Müllerian hormone levels and body weight, significantly reduced OHSS incidence without compromising clinical pregnancy rates, marking an important advance in stimulation safety [35].

A large retrospective cohort study of 1,435,108 oocyte retrievals using data from Japan's ART registry (2007–2015) identified high OHSS and hemoperitoneum risk associated with GnRH agonist protocols and fresh embryo transfers. The incidence of these complications has declined over time, in parallel with the reduced use of agonist protocols and increased adoption of frozen embryo transfer strategies [36].

4.2.5 Conclusion

OHSS remains a significant iatrogenic complication of controlled ovarian stimulation, particularly in patients triggered with hCG and those with identifiable risk factors such as PCOS or a history of OHSS. The cornerstone of prevention lies in individual risk assessment and tailored stimulation protocols. Use of GnRH antagonist protocols, with final oocyte maturation triggered by a GnRH agonist (alone or with low-dose hCG), is among the most effective strategies.

Additional interventions include the cryopreservation of embryos, metformin for PCOS patients, cabergoline, aspirin, and IV calcium, each showing promise in reducing OHSS rates without negatively impacting reproductive outcomes. Novel agents such as kisspeptin and the tailored use of follitropin delta represent exciting directions in OHSS prevention.

Given the associations between OHSS and adverse perinatal outcomes like low birth weight and preterm delivery, there is a strong imperative for its elimination. The future lies in OHSS-free clinics achieved through early identification of high-risk individuals and the implementation of individualized, evidence-based protocols for stimulation and prevention.

References

1. Papanikolaou EG, Pozzobon C, Kolibianakis EM, Camus M, Tournaye H, Fatemi HM, Van Steirteghem A, Devroey P. Incidence and prediction of ovarian hyperstimulation syndrome in women undergoing gonadotro-

pin releasing hormone antagonist in vitro fertilization cycles. Fertil Steril. 2006;

2. Navot D, Relou A, Birkenfield A, Rabinowitz R, Brzezinski A, MargaliothE J. Risk factors and prognostic variables in the ovarian hyperstimulation syndrome. Am J Obstet Gynecol. 1988;159:210–5.
3. Geva E, Jaffe RE. Role of vascular endothelial growth factor in ovarian physiology and pathology. Fertil Steril. 2000;74:429–38.
4. Soares SR. Etiology of OHSS and use of dopamine agonists. Fertil Steril. 2012;97(3):517–22.
5. Shmorgun D, Claman P, Gysler M, et al. Joint society of obstetricians and gynaecologists of Canada-Canadian fertility and andrology society clinical practice guidelines Committee. The diagnosis and management of ovarian hyperstimulation syndrome: no. 268, 2011. Int J Gynaecol Obstet. 2012;116:268–73.
6. Humaidan P, Nelson SM, Devroey P, Coddington CC, Schwartz LB, Gordon K, Frattarelli JL, Tarlatzis BC, Fatemi HM, Lutjen P, Stegmann BJ. Ovarian hyperstimulation syndrome: review and new classification criteria for reporting in clinical trials. Hum Reprod. 2016;31(9):1997–2004. https://doi.org/10.1093/humrep/dew149. Epub 2016 Jun 23
7. Lee KH, Kim SH, Jee BC, Kim YJ, Suh CS, Kim KC, Lee WD. Comparison of clinical characteristics between early and late patterns in hospitalized patients with ovarian hyperstimulation syndrome. Fertil Steril. 2010;93(7):2274–80.
8. Humaidan P, Quartarolo J, Papanikolaou EG. Preventing ovarian hyperstimulation syndrome: guidance for the clinician. Fertil Steril. 2010;94:389–400.
9. Delvigne A, Rozenberg S. Review of clinical course and treatment of ovarian hyperstimulation syndrome(OHSS). Hum Reprod Update. 2003;9:77–96.
10. Delvigne A, Kostyla K, Murillo D, Van Hoeck J, Rozenberg S. Oocyte quality and IVF outcome after coasting to prevent ovarian hyperstimulation syndrome. Int J Fertil Womens Med. 2003;48(1):25–31.
11. Navot D, Bergh PA, Laufer N. Ovarian hyperstimulation syndrome in novel reproductive technologies: prevention and treatment. Fertil Steril. 1992;58:249–61.
12. Asch RH, Li HP, Balmaceda JP, Weckstein LN, Stone SC. Severe ovarian hyperstimulation syndrome in assisted reproductive technology: definition of high risk groups. Hum Reprod. 1991;6(10):1395–9.
13. Enskog A, Henriksson M, Unander M, Nilsson L, Brännström M. Prospective study of the clinical and laboratory parameters of patients in whom ovarian hyperstimulation syndrome developed during controlled ovarian hyperstimulation for in vitro fertilization. Fertil Steril. 1999;71(5):808–14.

14. Luke B, Brown MB, Morbeck DE, Hudson SB, Coddington CC, Stern JE. Factors associated with ovarian hyperstimulation syndrome(OHSS) and its effect on assisted reproductive technology (ART) treatment and outcome. Fertil Steril. 2009;94:1399–404.
15. Semrl N, De Vos M, Blockeel C. The dark side of random-start ovarian stimulation: ovarian hyperstimulation syndrome due to inadvertent pregnancy. Reprod Biomed Online. 2024;49(4):104121.
16. Practice Committee of the American Society for Reproductive Medicine. Prevention of moderate and severe ovarian hyperstimulation syndrome: a guideline. Fertil Steril. 2024;121(2):230–45.
17. Grossman LC, et al. The pathophysiology of ovarian hyperstimulation syndrome: an unrecognized compartment syndrome. Fertil Steril. 2010;94(4):1392–8.
18. Abbara A, Jayasena CN, Christopoulos G, Narayanaswamy S, Izzi-Engbeaya C, Nijher GM, Comninos AN, Peters D, Buckley A, Ratnasabapathy R, et al. Efficacy of Kisspeptin-54 to trigger oocyte maturation in women at high risk of ovarian Hyperstimulation syndrome (OHSS)during in vitro fertilization (IVF) therapy. J Clin Endocrinol Metab. 2015;100:3322–31.
19. Ruohonen ST, Poutanen M, Tena-Sempere M. Role of kisspeptins in the control of the hypothalamic-pituitary-ovarian axis: old dogmas and new challenges. Fertil Steril. 2020;114(3):465–74.
20. Kwik M, Maxwell E. Pathophysiology, treatment and prevention of ovarian hyperstimulation syndrome. Curr Opin Obstet Gynecol. 2016;28(4):236–41.
21. Check JH, Choe JK, Nazari A. Hyperreactio luteinalis despite the absence of a corpus luteum and suppressed follicle stimulating concentrations in a triplet pregnancy. Hum Reprod. 2000;15:1043–5.
22. Ludwig M, Gembruch U, Bauer O, Diedrich K. Ovarian hyperstimulation syndrome (OHSS) in a spontaneous pregnancy with fetal and placental triploidy: information about the general pathophysiology of OHSS. Hum Reprod. 1998;13:2082–7.
23. Nappi RG, Di Nero E, D'Aries AP, Nappi L. Natural pregnancy in hypothyroid woman complicated by spontaneous ovarian hyperstimulation syndrome. Am J Obstet Gynecol. 1998;178:610–1.
24. DiCarlo C, Bruno PA, Cirillo D, Morgera R, Pellicano M, Nappi C. Increased concentrations of renin, aldosterone and Ca^{125} in a case of spontaneous, recurrent, familial, severe ovarian hyperstimulation syndrome. Hum Reprod. 1997;12:2115–7.
25. Schirmer DA III, Kulkarni AD, Zhang Y, Kawwass JF, Boulet SL, Kissin DM. Ovarian hyperstimulation syndrome after assisted reproductive technologies: trends, predictors, and pregnancy outcomes. Fertil Steril. 2020;114(3):567–78.

26. Blockeel C, Campbell A, Coticchio G, Esler J, Garcia-Velasco JA, Santulli P, Pinborg A. Should we still perform fresh embryo transfers in ART? Hum Reprod. 2019;34(12):2319–29.
27. Papanikolaou EG, Tournaye H, Verpoest W, Camus M, Vernaeve V, Van Steirteghem A, Devroey P. Early and late ovarian hyperstimulation syndrome: early pregnancy outcome and profile. Hum Reprod. 2005;20(3):636–41. https://doi.org/10.1093/humrep/deh638.
28. Yakovenko SA, Zorina IV, Dmitrieva NV, Sivozhelezov VS, Dyakonov SA. Intravenous administration of calcium in ovarian hyperstimulation syndrome (OHSS) prevention. Fertil Steril. 2011;96(3):S20.
29. Varnagy A, Bodis J, Manfai Z, Wilhelm F, Busznyak C, Koppan M. Low-dose aspirin therapy to prevent ovarian hyperstimulation syndrome. Fertil Steril. 2010;93:2281–4.
30. Revelli A, Dolfin E, Gennarelli G, Lantieri T, Massobrio M, Holte JG, et al. Low-dose acetylsalicylic acid plus prednisolone as an adjuvant treatment in IVF: a prospective, randomized study. Fertil Steril. 2008;90:1685–91.
31. Palomba S, Falbo A, La Sala GB. Effects of metformin in women with polycystic ovary syndrome treated with gonadotrophins for in vitro fertilisation and intracytoplasmic sperm injection cycles: a systematic review and meta-analysis of randomised controlled trials. BJOG. 2013;120:267–76.
32. Huang X, Wang P, Tal R, Lv F, Li Y, Zhang X. A systematic review and meta-analysis of metformin among patients with polycystic ovary syndrome undergoing assisted reproductive technology procedures. Int J Gynaecol Obstet. 2015;131:111–6.
33. Lainas GT, Kolibianakis EM, Sfontouris IA, Zorzovilis IZ, Petsas GK, Lainas TG, Tarlatzis BC. Pregnancy and neonatal outcomes following luteal GnRH antagonist administration in patients with severe early OHSS. Hum Reprod. 2013;28(7):1929–42. https://doi.org/10.1093/humrep/dct114.
34. Leitao VM, Moroni RM, Seko LM, Nastri CO, Martins WP. Cabergoline for the prevention of ovarian hyperstimulation syndrome: systematic review and meta-analysis of randomized controlled trials. Fertil Steril. 2014;101:664–75.
35. Ishihara O, et al. Reduction in Ohss incidence in Japanese Ivf/Icsi patients when applying individualized dosing with Follitropin Delta. Fertil Steril. 2020;114(3):e457.
36. Kuroda K, Nagai S, Ikemoto Y, Matsumura Y, Ochiai A, Nojiri S, Itakura A, Sugiyama R. Incidences and risk factors of moderate-to-severe ovarian hyperstimulation syndrome and severe hemoperitoneum in 1,435,108 oocyte retrievals. Reprod Biomed Online. 2021;42(1):125–32.

Role of Counseling in an OHSS-Free Clinic

5

Daniel S. Seidman and Liron Seidman

5.1 Introduction

Ovarian hyperstimulation syndrome (OHSS) is a major risk of fertility treatments and a major concern for patients [1]. As patients must be well informed regarding the possible risks of IVF treatment, they must also be reassured regarding the physician's responsibility for prevention and improved ability in caring for this serious complication.

Counseling plays a crucial role in informing patients about the risks and prevention strategies of OHSS (Table 5.1). This chapter explores strategies to enhance our counseling efforts with the underlying goal of achieving an OHSS-free clinic.

D. S. Seidman · L. Seidman (✉)
Department of Obstetrics and Gynecology, The Chaim Sheba Medical Center, Tel-Hashomer, Israel and The Faculty of Medical & Health Sciences, Tel Aviv University, Tel Aviv, Israel
e-mail: dseidman@post.tau.ac.il

G. N. Allahbadia et al. (eds.), *Ovarian Hyperstimulation Syndrome (OHSS) Free Clinic*, https://doi.org/10.1007/978-981-95-3289-6_5

Table 5.1 How counseling plays a crucial role in informing patients about the risks and prevention strategies of ovarian hyperstimulation syndrome (OHSS)

Aspect	Description	Importance
Risk awareness	Inform patients about their individual risk factors for OHSS	Helps patients understand their personal risk level
Early intervention	Identify high-risk patients and implement preventive strategies	Allows for proactive management and risk reduction
Informed decision-making	Provide information on treatment options and potential risks	Empowers patients to actively participate in their care plan
Symptom awareness	Educate patients about signs and symptoms of OHSS	Enables early recognition and timely medical attention
Preventive strategies	Discuss various preventive measures and modified protocols	Helps reduce the likelihood of OHSS occurrence
Psychological preparation	Address potential anxiety and prepare patients mentally	Improves patient coping and reduces stress
Compliance with monitoring	Emphasize the importance of regular check-ups and tests	Ensures timely detection of OHSS development
Discussion of alternatives	Present alternative approaches for high-risk cases	Provides options to minimize OHSS risk while pursuing treatment

5.2 Risk Awareness

In fertility clinics, counseling has a pivotal role in educating patients about OHSS, especially among patients undergoing assisted reproductive technology (ART). One of the key components of counseling is informing patients about the factors that increase their likelihood of developing OHSS. Risk awareness is crucial for patients undergoing IVF who have an increased likelihood of developing OHSS. This includes patients with elevated anti-Müllerian hormone (AMH) levels, polycystic ovary syndrome (PCOS), and those expected to have high oocyte yields [1].

By helping patients recognize these risk factors, they become better equipped to make informed decisions about their fertility treatment options.

When providing counseling, it should be emphasized that while risk factors exist,

ovarian stimulation protocols based on individual risk factors and ovarian reserve testing should be offered and discussed. The rationale for using GnRH antagonist protocols over GnRH agonist protocols in high-risk cases should be explained. To avoid unnecessary disappointment, patients should be prepared for the possibility that a fresh embryo transfer will not be performed immediately after ovum aspiration if oocyte yield is high or a GnRH agonist trigger is used.

5.3 Prevention Strategies

Counseling should offer patients valuable insights into prevention strategies for OHSS, providing them with reassurance that their healthcare providers are aware of their risks and are implementing effective measures to reduce the likelihood of OHSS occurring. For instance, clinicians can discuss the benefits of using lower-dose gonadotropin protocols, switching to GnRH agonist triggers instead of hCG, or employing a "freeze-all" strategy where embryos are frozen for transfer at a later time.

Early intervention plays a major role in current practice [2]. By identifying high-risk patients early through counseling, clinicians can individualize gonadotropin dosing, implement preventive strategies, and modify treatment protocols before starting ovarian stimulation. The efficacy and safety of an individualized fixed daily dose of gonadotropins, based on body weight and AMH, have been established in randomized controlled trials (RCTs) using a GnRH antagonist protocol and, more recently, GnRH agonist protocols [3].

Patients must be informed of these interventions as proven means that can significantly reduce the risk of OHSS, particularly in patients who are more vulnerable due to their underlying risk factors. The use of medical preventive measures like administering Cabergoline after ovum pickup should be explained, stressing common side effects like constipation and disturbed sleep. Proper counseling ensures that patients fully understand the benefits of these contemporary approaches, empowering them to take part in choosing the best preventive measures.

Counseling is essential in empowering patients to make informed choices about their treatment plans. By offering clear and comprehensive explanations of the risks and benefits associated with each option, clinicians enable patients to actively engage in the decision-making process regarding their fertility treatment. Patients can feel more confident in their choices when they understand the full scope of the preventive strategies available, which can lead to better outcomes and reduced anxiety.

5.4 Informed Decision-Making

Patients are often self-educated when first attending the IVF clinic. The abundance of information provided by friends and social networks, however, may be misleading or disproportional at times, and even cause undue concern [4]. Increased anxiety was found to be prevalent among infertile women and may influence decision-making [5].

Informed decision-making may alleviate some of the patients' concerns regarding OHSS. It is important to discuss the benefits and risks of proceeding with treatment versus alternative approaches, e.g., cycle cancellation or a freeze-all strategy. Involving patients in the decision-making process regarding preventive measures and management options has become part of everyday patient counseling.

A small multicenter discrete choice experiment recently found among women at higher risk of OHSS that the likelihood of developing OHSS plays a significant role in shaping their preference for IVF treatment [6]. The study revealed that many women are willing to accept trade-offs, such as dealing with side effects, higher costs, or a reduced chance of pregnancy, in exchange for a lower risk of OHSS [6].

Counseling provides patients with the necessary information to make informed decisions about their treatment options and potential risks. This empowers patients to actively participate in their care plan. Patients should be educated about the signs and symptoms of OHSS, enabling them to recognize early warning signs and seek timely medical attention if needed.

5.5 Reassurance

Patients should be made aware that, although OHSS remains a potential risk, modern IVF clinics have achieved dramatic strides, and an OHSS-free clinic is no longer a dream [7]. Patients should be informed that through reducing or eliminating the use of hCG and using GnRH agonist-triggered GnRH antagonist cycles, OHSS has been practically eliminated. Cryopreservation of oocytes or embryos is now routinely practiced and guarantees good success rates when such treatment strategies are implemented. Counseling sessions can be used to discuss various preventive measures, such as individualized gonadotropin dosing and the use of cabergoline.

Patients should be informed about the importance of regular monitoring during ovarian stimulation, including ultrasound and hormone level checks, to assess their risk of OHSS throughout the treatment cycle. They should be made aware that, through careful monitoring, the physician can identify an increased ovarian response and ensure a safe outcome by modifying gonadotropin doses and using a GnRH agonist trigger.

5.6 Monitoring, Follow-Up, and Symptom Awareness

It is important during a clinic consultation not to miss the opportunity to educate patients about the signs and symptoms of OHSS, emphasizing the importance of early reporting. The spectrum of OHSS severity and potential complications should be clearly discussed. Possible management strategies, if OHSS develops, must be explained, including increased fluid intake and close monitoring for mild-to-moderate cases. The potential need for cryopreservation of all embryos in severe cases of OHSS or even a possible cycle cancellation in extreme situations must be noted, especially for patients at risk or during a GnRH agonist cycle.

It is important for patients undergoing such treatments to be aware of the early and late symptoms of OHSS and to report them to their physician as soon as they occur, as the condition can range from mild to severe. Early symptoms of OHSS typically include mild to moderate abdominal bloating or swelling, accompanied by discomfort or pain in the lower abdomen. Some patients may experience mild nausea, vomiting, and diarrhea. Additionally, sudden weight gain, typically more than 2.2 pounds (or 1 kg) in a day, may also occur. Another early sign to watch for is an increase in urination. These symptoms should be reported to the physician, as they could indicate the onset of OHSS, and early intervention can help prevent the condition from worsening.

As OHSS progresses, more severe symptoms can develop, and these require urgent medical attention. Severe abdominal pain or bloating, rapid weight gain (more than 2 pounds or 1 kg per day), and a noticeable decrease in urination despite adequate fluid intake are concerning signs. Patients may also experience more intense nausea and vomiting, along with shortness of breath or difficulty breathing, which can indicate fluid accumulation in the chest or abdomen. Dark urine, dizziness, or lightheadedness are also warning signs of severe OHSS. In some cases, the patient may experience swelling in the legs or arms, severe chest pain, or palpitations, which could indicate the formation of blood clots. These severe symptoms are rare but can be life-threatening, requiring hospitalization.

Patients must be instructed that if any of the symptoms mentioned above appear, it is crucial that they contact their physician without delay for appropriate care.

When consulting the patient, the importance of regular monitoring during and after stimulation must be emphasized. The clinic's protocol for follow-up and when to seek immediate medical attention should always be outlined to the patient.

5.7 Fear of OHSS

Concern regarding the risk of developing OHSS during IVF is common among women undergoing fertility treatments. Patients are often made aware, through friends and family, as well as social media, of the symptoms of OHSS, ranging from abdominal discomfort and fluid retention to, in rare cases, serious complications requiring hospitalization. This fear is related not only to potential physical discomfort but also to concerns about how OHSS might affect the success of the IVF cycle.

Several factors contribute to this fear. Uncertainty and loss of control are significant sources of anxiety, as women undergoing IVF already face a challenging and emotionally taxing process. The possibility of developing OHSS adds another layer of unpredictability, leaving women concerned about how their bodies will respond to treatment. Additionally, the potential health risks associated with OHSS, such as blood clots, kidney problems, or fluid in the lungs, can be frightening, even though severe cases are rare.

For many women, the fear of OHSS is compounded by the possibility of treatment delays. Moderate to severe OHSS can require postponing embryo transfer, which can be emotionally distressing for women who are eager to achieve pregnancy. This extended timeline can add further psychological pressure. Women with a history of OHSS or those who know others who have experienced it may be particularly anxious about facing the condition themselves.

Psychologically, the fear of OHSS can intensify the already heavy burden of fertility treatments, leading to increased anxiety and stress. This fear can influence decision-making, with some women opting for more conservative treatment approaches to avoid OHSS, even though it may affect their overall chances of success.

Addressing these fears begins with education and counseling. When women are well informed about the risks of OHSS and the preventive strategies available, they can feel more in control. Counseling with fertility specialists or mental health professionals can also help alleviate fears by providing a deeper understanding of the condition and personalized guidance on managing anxiety.

Personalized treatment plans play a crucial role in reducing the risk of OHSS and alleviating fear [1]. By tailoring protocols to each patient's individual risk factors, such as opting for lower-dose stimulation or using alternative ovulation triggers, doctors can reassure patients that their treatment is designed to minimize the likelihood of OHSS. This individualized approach, combined with close monitoring throughout the IVF cycle, can help women feel more secure, knowing that early signs of OHSS will be promptly addressed.

Lastly, having a support network is essential for coping with the emotional stress of IVF and the fear of OHSS. Whether through partners, family, friends, or support groups, emotional support can help women feel less isolated in their experience and more confident in managing their fears.

In summary, while the fear of OHSS is valid, it can be mitigated through education, personalized care, psychological support, and vigilant medical monitoring. These strategies not only help women feel more in control of their fertility journey but also improve their emotional well-being during the treatment process.

5.8 Emotional Support

Counseling provides essential emotional support to patients who may be anxious or fearful about the potential complications of OHSS. Fertility treatments can be emotionally taxing, and the possibility of developing OHSS adds an additional layer of stress [8]. The assessment of psychological disorders and stress hormone dysregulation should not be overlooked in infertile women seeking IVF treatment [5]. Through counseling, patients receive not only medical information but also reassurance and guidance on managing their emotional health throughout the process. Fertility caregivers can reassure couples that current research shows that a woman's biological response to ovarian stimulation is not influenced by either partner's level of psychological distress [9].

Providing psychological preparation by discussing the potential risks and management strategies, counseling can help alleviate anxiety and prepare patients mentally for the possibility of OHSS. In high-risk cases, counseling provides an opportunity to discuss alternative approaches, such as cycle cancellation or freeze-all strategies, to minimize OHSS risk.

Psychological support can be provided for women who are fearful of developing OHSS during IVF by individual counseling or therapy. In these sessions, women can address their specific concerns and explore the emotional toll that fertility treatments and the possibility of OHSS can take. Cognitive-behavioral therapy (CBT) is particularly useful for helping women manage anxiety by providing tools to reframe negative thoughts and reduce stress. Counseling offers a safe space to discuss fears openly, and therapists can offer techniques to manage the emotional burden of treatment.

Another essential form of support comes from education and clear communication. When women are well informed about OHSS, its risks, and the measures in place to prevent it, they tend to feel more in control of their treatment and less fearful. Healthcare providers can educate patients about the careful monitoring protocols and tailored medication plans designed to minimize the risk of OHSS. This transparency reassures patients and alleviates much of the anxiety associated with the unknown aspects of treatment.

Support groups, whether in-person or online, offer emotional comfort by allowing women to connect with others going through similar experiences. Sharing personal stories and advice with others who understand the emotional and physical toll of fertility treatment can reduce feelings of isolation and fear. Support groups foster a sense of community and shared understanding, which can be invaluable during emotionally challenging times.

Mindfulness and stress-reduction techniques are also highly effective for managing the anxiety associated with fertility treatments and the risk of OHSS. Practices like meditation, deep breathing, and yoga help women relax and improve their emotional resilience. Many fertility clinics encourage patients to engage in mindfulness-based stress reduction (MBSR) programs to better cope with the stresses of the treatment journey.

The involvement of partners and family members is another key element of psychological support. Having loved ones present during consultations or treatments can provide emotional reassurance, helping to alleviate fear and share the burden of stress. Partners, in particular, can be a source of comfort and emotional strength, making the IVF process feel more like a joint effort.

Lastly, open communication with the medical team and personalized care are essential for easing anxiety. When patients feel heard, understood, and involved in their treatment plans, they are more likely to trust the process and feel reassured. Regular updates on the patient's condition and careful monitoring throughout the IVF cycle can help alleviate fears and build confidence in the treatment approach.

By integrating these strategies—counseling, education, support groups, mindfulness, involvement of loved ones, and open communication with the healthcare team—clinics can provide comprehensive psychological support to help women manage their fears about OHSS and enhance their emotional well-being throughout their IVF journey.

5.9 Social Media

Social media has become an influential platform for women undergoing IVF, especially in relation to concerns about OHSS [10]. It serves as a source of both information and emotional support, helping women navigate their IVF journeys. Fertility clinics, doctors, and patient advocacy groups often use platforms like Instagram, Facebook, and Twitter to share critical information about the risks, symptoms, and prevention of OHSS [11]. Through social media posts, blogs, and videos, complex medical concepts surrounding OHSS are made accessible to a broader audience, empowering patients with knowledge and helping them make informed decisions about their treatment.

Another key aspect of social media is the peer support it offers. Many women share their personal IVF journeys, including experiences with OHSS, on platforms such as Facebook groups, Reddit threads, or Instagram accounts. These firsthand stories can provide emotional comfort and help others feel less alone in their fertility struggles. Online support groups allow patients to exchange advice, share symptoms, and offer encouragement. This peer-to-peer interaction fosters a sense of community and shared understanding, which can be particularly valuable in dealing with the emotional stresses of fertility treatments [10, 11].

However, the widespread availability of information on social media also has its downsides. Not all the content shared is accurate or evidence-based, and misinformation about OHSS can spread quickly. Stories of severe cases or exaggerated outcomes can heighten anxiety among IVF patients, leading to unnecessary fear. For instance, anecdotal stories or advice based on one person's experience may not be applicable to others but can still influence how they perceive their risk. It is essential for patients to critically evaluate the information they encounter online and consult their fertility specialists for guidance rather than relying solely on social media.

The emotional impact of social media can be both positive and negative. While it can be encouraging to see others successfully navigate their IVF treatments, constant exposure to posts about complications, failed cycles, or others' successes can cause emotional stress or lead to unrealistic comparisons. This can amplify anxiety, especially for women who are already concerned about complications like OHSS. It is important for patients to maintain a balanced perspective when using social media, recognizing that each IVF journey is unique.

Influencers and fertility specialists play a pivotal role in how OHSS is discussed online. Many specialists use their platforms to dispel myths, provide accurate information, and offer tips for managing the risk of OHSS. Influencers who have personally experienced IVF can offer emotional support and share their strategies for coping with the physical and psychological aspects of the process. These voices help build a supportive and informed online community, fostering both education and empathy for those navigating fertility challenges [11].

In conclusion, while social media can be a valuable resource for information and emotional support regarding OHSS, it should be used cautiously. Fertility experts should ensure that their patients' medical decisions are guided by their professional consultation and that they rely on social media only as a supplementary tool for connection and shared experience, rather than a primary source of information.

5.10 Artificial Intelligence (AI) and Smart Apps

New technology and artificial intelligence (AI) may transform the way OHSS is managed in IVF treatments [12–15]. One of the most significant applications of AI is in predictive modeling, where machine learning algorithms analyze vast amounts of patient data—such as age, hormonal levels, ovarian reserve markers (AMH, AFC), and response to previous treatments—to predict which patients are at the highest risk of developing OHSS [13]. These AI-driven models can detect patterns in data that might not be obvious through traditional methods, allowing for earlier identification of high-risk patients [14]. This enables healthcare providers to tailor treatments more effectively, helping to mitigate the risk of OHSS while optimizing IVF success rates [13, 15].

In addition to prediction, AI is also instrumental in personalizing treatment protocols [14]. For instance, by analyzing real-time data on a patient's hormonal responses and follicular development during the IVF cycle, AI algorithms can recommend specific dosages of gonadotropins or suggest alternative ovulation triggers, such as using a GnRH agonist instead of hCG, to lower the chances of OHSS. This level of personalization allows for a more controlled ovarian stimulation process, reducing the risk of overstimulation while maintaining the likelihood of a successful outcome.

Smartphone-based apps that incorporate AI for self-monitoring are another technological advancement helping to manage OHSS risk [15]. These apps can collect patient-reported symptoms, such as bloating or abdominal pain, and track relevant health data like weight changes. AI algorithms within the apps can analyze this data to assess a patient's risk of developing OHSS and alert both the patient and healthcare providers to any warning signs. This allows for early intervention, which is crucial in preventing moderate cases of OHSS from progressing into more severe forms. By empowering patients to self-monitor, these apps enhance the overall safety and efficacy of IVF treatments [15].

A recent study described the development of multiphase predictive models for OHSS using retrospective big data to aid physicians in assessing and making clinical decisions [15]. These models reliably identify patients at high risk of OHSS. The investigators created a user-friendly smartphone app designed for the personalized management of women at risk of moderate to severe OHSS. By integrating this self-monitoring app, high-risk patients can be empowered to engage in early detection and management of the condition. The combination of predictive models and the app improves management strategies for patients at risk of OHSS, offering efficient support for personalized care. Ongoing prospective validation of both the model and the app is needed to further assess their clinical effectiveness and utility [15].

One key advantage of this predictive-model-based app is its ability to provide individualized risk assessments for each woman at specific consultation points [15]. This allows for tailored clinical decisions to be made accordingly. Given that assisted reproductive care is often limited to urban areas, women in low-income or remote settings with limited healthcare access can especially benefit from the app's early OHSS risk alerts. By automatically retrieving parameter values from clinical databases, the app generates a personalized risk score. Based on this predictive risk, physicians can implement optimal strategies to mitigate OHSS risk in subsequent stages of treatment. For those identified as high-risk, strict follow-up and careful self-monitoring are recommended.

Through the app's self-monitoring module, patients become more aware of OHSS-related symptoms such as nausea, abdominal distension, and pain, and are prompted to schedule follow-up visits if the app indicates increased risk [15]. This proactive monitoring reduces the likelihood of delayed diagnosis and management of OHSS. Overall, this app has the potential to significantly enhance the management of women at risk for OHSS and improve the safety of assisted reproductive treatments. However, further prospective studies are needed to confirm its effectiveness and performance in clinical settings [15].

Real-time monitoring systems, powered by AI, further support clinicians by continuously tracking a patient's hormone levels and follicle development throughout the IVF cycle [14]. These systems provide real-time data that can help doctors adjust treatment protocols dynamically, ensuring a safe and well-regulated process. For example, if the AI detects abnormal hormone responses or excessive follicular growth, it can flag the need to adjust medication or the timing of ovulation triggers to prevent OHSS.

Finally, AI's role in analyzing genetic data offers promising insights into genetic predispositions that may increase a patient's risk for OHSS. By evaluating genetic variants, such as those in the FSH receptor or VEGF pathway, AI systems can help identify patients who are genetically more susceptible to OHSS. This enables even more precise customization of fertility treatments, tailored to the genetic makeup of the individual, which can further reduce the risk of OHSS.

In summary, AI and smart apps are significantly improving our ability to responsibly consult on and manage OHSS in IVF by providing more accurate risk prediction, personalized treatment plans, real-time monitoring, and self-management tools. As AI technology continues to advance, it promises to make IVF treatments safer, more efficient, and more accessible to patients at risk of OHSS.

5.11 Conclusions

Counseling is a crucial component in managing the risk of OHSS. It informs patients about risk factors, introduces prevention strategies, supports informed decision-making, provides emotional reassurance, and emphasizes the importance of close monitoring throughout the fertility treatment journey. This comprehensive approach ensures that patients are better prepared, both physically and emotionally, to navigate the challenges of

OHSS prevention and treatment. By ensuring patients are educated on recognizing early signs of OHSS and are well advised on when to seek medical help, clinicians can intervene early to prevent the condition from worsening, thereby improving patient safety and outcomes.

References

1. Practice Committee of the American Society for Reproductive Medicine. Prevention of moderate and severe ovarian hyperstimulation syndrome: a guideline. Fertil Steril. 2024;121(2):230–45.
2. Nelson SM, Shaw M, Alrashid K, Anderson RA. Individualized dosing of follitropin delta affects live birth and safety in in vitro fertilization treatment: an individual participant data meta-analysis of randomized controlled trials. Fertil Steril. 2024;S0015-0282(24):00453–9.
3. Lobo R, Soerdal T, Ekerhovd E, Cohlen B, Porcu E, Schenk M, Shufaro Y, Smeenk J, Suerdieck MB, Pinton P, Pinborg A, Investigators BEYOND. BEYOND: a randomized controlled trial comparing efficacy and safety of individualized follitropin delta dosing in a GnRH agonist versus antagonist protocol during the first ovarian stimulation cycle. Hum Reprod. 2024;9:deae092.
4. Galiano V, Orvieto R, Machtinger R, Nahum R, Garzia E, Sulpizio P, Marconi AM, Seidman D. "Add-Ons" for assisted reproductive technology: do patients get honest information from fertility clinics' websites? Reprod Sci. 2021;28(12):3466–72.
5. Chai Y, Li Q, Wang Y, Niu B, Chen H, Fan T, Ke X, Zou H. Cortisol dysregulation in anxiety infertile women and the influence on IVF treatment outcome. Front Endocrinol (Lausanne). 2023;14:1107765.
6. Braam SC, de Bruin JP, Mol BWJ, van Wely M. The perspective of women with an increased risk of OHSS regarding the safety and burden of IVF: a discrete choice experiment. Hum Reprod Open. 2020;2020(2):hoz034.
7. Banker M, Garcia-Velasco JA. Revisiting ovarian hyper stimulation syndrome: towards OHSS free clinic. J Hum Reprod Sci. 2015;8(1):13–7.
8. Zanettoullis AT, Mastorakos G, Vakas P, Vlahos N, Valsamakis G. Effect of stress on each of the stages of the IVF procedure: a systematic review. Int J Mol Sci. 2024;25(2):726.
9. Donarelli Z, Lo Coco G, Gullo S, Marino A, Volpes A, Salerno L, Allegra A. Infertility-related stress, anxiety and ovarian stimulation: can couples be reassured about the effects of psychological factors on biological responses to assisted reproductive technology? Reprod Biomed Soc Online. 2016;3:16–23.

10. Peyser A, Goldstein L, Mullin C, Goldman RH. Fertility education: what's trending on Instagram. Fertil Res Pract. 2021;7(1):3.
11. Miller N, Pundak C, Cohen G, Issakov G, Gluska H, Gandelsman E, Frishman EK, David L, Bookstein SP, Goldenberg J, Wiser A. Can social support on Facebook influence fertility outcomes? Reprod Sci. 2022;29(1):212–9.
12. Guo X, Zhan H, Zhang X, Pang Y, Xu H, Zhang B, Lao K, Ding P, Wang Y, Han L. Predictive models for starting dose of gonadotropin in controlled ovarian hyperstimulation: review and progress update. Hum Fertil (Camb). 2023;26(6):1609–16.
13. Ziaee A, Khosravi H, Sadeghi T, Ahmed I, Mahmoudinia M. Prediction of complicated ovarian hyperstimulation syndrome in assisted reproductive treatment through artificial intelligence. medRxiv 2024.04.17.24305980.
14. AlSaad R, Abd-Alrazaq A, Choucair F, Ahmed A, Aziz S, Sheikh J. Harnessing artificial intelligence to predict ovarian stimulation outcomes in in vitro fertilization: scoping review. J Med Internet Res. 2024;26:e53396.
15. Cao M, Liu Z, Lin Y, Luo Y, Li S, Huang Q, Liu H, Liu J. A personalized management approach of OHSS: development of a multiphase prediction model and smartphone-based app. Front Endocrinol (Lausanne). 2022;13:911225.

Role of Ovarian Markers in the Prevention of OHSS

6

Salvatore Scaglione and Andrea Borini

6.1 Rationale

The increasing utilization of assisted reproductive technologies (ART) has underscored the critical need to mitigate the risks associated with ovarian hyperstimulation syndrome (OHSS), a potentially severe complication. Ovarian markers such as anti-Müllerian hormone (AMH) and antral follicle count (AFC) have become pivotal tools for predicting and preventing OHSS. These markers enable clinicians to stratify patients by risk before initiating ovarian stimulation, allowing for the customization of treatment protocols. This individualized approach significantly reduces the likelihood of OHSS, enhancing patient safety and treatment efficacy. "Role of Ovarian Markers in Prevention of OHSS" aims to provide a comprehensive overview of the current understanding and application of these ovarian markers in clinical practice. It synthesizes recent research findings, clinical case studies, and emerging therapeutic strategies to offer a detailed guide for fertility specialists. By exploring both established and novel preventive measures, this chapter seeks to improve clinical outcomes in ART, ensuring that treatments are both effective and safe for patients.

S. Scaglione · A. Borini (✉)
IVIRMA Global Research Alliance, Bologna, Italy
e-mail: andrea.borini@9puntobaby.it

G. N. Allahbadia et al. (eds.), *Ovarian Hyperstimulation Syndrome (OHSS) Free Clinic*, https://doi.org/10.1007/978-981-95-3289-6_6

Through this focused examination, the chapter aspires to advance the field of reproductive medicine, promoting evidence-based practices that prioritize patient well-being. It serves as an essential resource for clinicians, researchers, and healthcare professionals dedicated to optimizing fertility treatments and minimizing the risks associated with ovarian hyperstimulation.

6.2 Introduction

Ovarian hyperstimulation syndrome (OHSS) is a serious complication associated with assisted reproductive technologies (ART). OHSS can range from mild to severe forms, and in the most severe cases, it poses significant health risks, including respiratory issues, coagulopathies, and renal dysfunction. Therefore, preventing OHSS is a fundamental priority in fertility treatment management [1]. A crucial aspect of preventing OHSS is identifying patients at risk. Women with polycystic ovary syndrome (PCOS), for instance, have a higher incidence of OHSS due to the large number of follicles recruited during gonadotropin therapy [1]. Additionally, hormonal markers such as anti-Müllerian hormone (AMH) and antral follicle count (AFC) have been identified as reliable predictors of ovarian response and the risk of developing OHSS [1]. Recent studies have shown that elevated AMH levels are correlated with a higher risk of OHSS. Specifically, AMH values above 3.36 ng/mL are associated with a significantly increased risk of OHSS, with a sensitivity of 90.5% and specificity of 81.3%. The adoption of international standards for AMH measurement could facilitate its broader clinical applicability [2]. Preventing OHSS involves more than just identifying risk. Strategies such as modifying stimulation protocols, using GnRH antagonists instead of agonists, and individualizing gonadotropin doses based on ovarian reserve have shown promising results in lowering the incidence of OHSS [3]. Additional approaches include coasting, careful selection of ovulation trigger agents, and the use of agents such as dopamine agonists and metformin, to mitigate the risk of OHSS [4]. In summary, managing OHSS requires a multidimensional approach that includes pretreatment risk marker assessment, personalized stimulation protocols, and the implementation of evidence-based preventive strategies. Continuous refinement of these techniques promises to improve the safety and efficacy of fertility treatments while minimizing the risk of OHSS.

6.3 Clinical Discussion

Ovarian hyperstimulation syndrome (OHSS) is a serious iatrogenic complication of controlled ovarian stimulation (COS) commonly associated with assisted reproductive technologies (ART). OHSS is characterized by ovarian enlargement and fluid shifts from the intravascular to the third space, leading to symptoms ranging from mild discomfort to severe life-threatening conditions [5]. Preventing OHSS is crucial, and recent research highlights the importance of ovarian markers such as anti-Müllerian hormone (AMH) and antral follicle count (AFC) in predicting and preventing OHSS [4].

6.4 Pathophysiology of OHSS

The pathophysiology of OHSS is primarily linked to the exposure of human chorionic gonadotropin (hCG), which increases vascular endothelial growth factor (VEGF) secretion, leading to increased vascular permeability and fluid extravasation (Fig. 6.1) [6]. The two clinical forms of OHSS—early and late—are distinguished by their time of onset. Early OHSS occurs within 9 days of hCG administration, while late OHSS occurs more than 10 days after, often due to endogenous hCG from an implanting embryo [1].

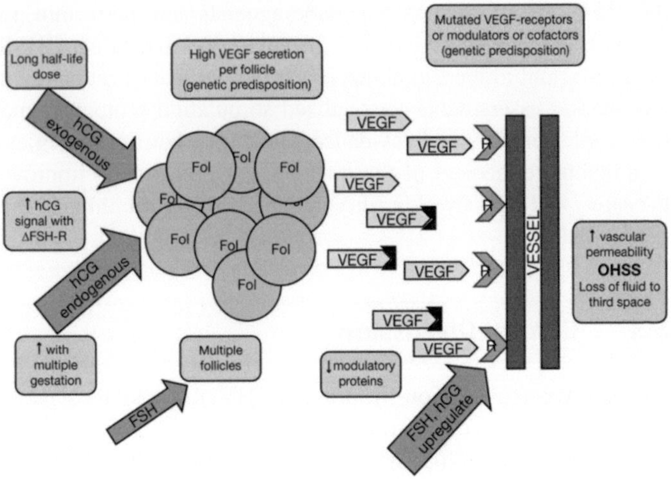

Fig. 6.1 The pathogenesis of OHSS

6.5 Risk Stratification and Ovarian Markers

Effective prevention of OHSS begins with identifying women at high risk. Key markers include:

1. *Anti-Müllerian hormone (AMH):* AMH is a reliable marker for predicting ovarian response. High pretreatment AMH levels are associated with an increased risk of OHSS.
2. *Antral follicle count (AFC):* AFC, assessed via ultrasound, provides an estimate of the ovarian reserve. A high AFC correlates with an increased risk of OHSS.

6.6 Preventive Strategies

6.6.1 Primary Prevention

1. *Individualized COS (iCOS):* Tailoring stimulation protocols based on ovarian markers such as AMH and AFC can help reduce the risk of OHSS. For instance, lower starting doses

of gonadotropins and adjusted stimulation regimens based on these markers can minimize excessive ovarian response [4].
2. *GnRH antagonist protocols:* Using GnRH antagonists instead of agonists can significantly reduce the risk of OHSS by preventing the initial ovarian hyperstimulation.
3. *Alternative ovulation triggers:* Replacing hCG with GnRH agonists for triggering ovulation has been shown to nearly eliminate the risk of OHSS in high-risk women, particularly when combined with cryopreservation of embryos.
4. *Adjunctive therapies:* Medications like metformin and dopamine agonists (e.g., cabergoline) have shown promise in reducing the incidence and severity of OHSS by modulating ovarian response and vascular permeability [7, 8].

6.6.2 Secondary Prevention

For women who exhibit signs of hyperstimulation during a cycle:

1. *Coasting:* Temporarily withholding gonadotropins while continuing GnRH antagonist administration until estradiol levels decrease can help mitigate the risk of OHSS.
2. *Cryopreservation of all embryos:* Freezing all embryos and delaying transfer to a subsequent cycle allows for the resolution of OHSS risk before pregnancy is attempted [9].

6.6.3 Emerging Therapies

Recent research has explored novel therapies such as vasopressin V1a receptor antagonists to inhibit VEGF secretion and prevent OHSS. Although still under investigation, these therapies hold potential for future clinical application. Preventing OHSS requires a multifaceted approach that includes risk stratification using ovarian markers, individualized treatment protocols, and both primary and secondary preventive strategies [10]. By incorporating markers like AMH and AFC into clinical practice, alongside emerging therapies, the incidence of OHSS can be significantly reduced, enhancing the safety and effectiveness of assisted reproductive technologies [9].

6.6.4 Case Studies

Early studies suggested that OHSS occurred in 20–33% of ART cycles, with moderate and severe OHSS in 3–8% of cycles when hCG was the primary option for oocyte maturation [11]. Techniques to reduce OHSS risks, such as GnRH antagonist protocols, GnRH agonist triggers, and the use of metformin and dopamine agonists, have been in use for 15–20 years [12]. Despite these advancements, OHSS remains a concern, with hospitalization rates stabilizing between 2008 and 2014 [12]. Recent case studies emphasize the pivotal role of ovarian markers in the prevention of ovarian hyperstimulation syndrome (OHSS). One significant study conducted in 2023 involved a high-risk patient with elevated anti-Müllerian hormone (AMH) levels and high antral follicle count (AFC). By adjusting the stimulation protocol based on these markers and utilizing a GnRH agonist trigger instead of hCG, the development of severe OHSS was effectively prevented. Additionally, cabergoline was administered to inhibit VEGF-mediated vascular permeability, further reducing the risk [13]. Another case study explored the use of individualized controlled ovarian stimulation (iCOS) protocols tailored to AMH and AFC levels. This approach not only minimized the risk of OHSS but also optimized the number of retrieved oocytes and improved pregnancy outcomes. The incorporation of adjunctive therapies, such as metformin, further demonstrated the effectiveness of these personalized strategies in clinical practice [13]. A comprehensive review highlighted multiple interventions, including the use of GnRH antagonists and the strategic timing of ovulation triggers, which have been shown to significantly reduce the incidence of OHSS in patients identified as high-risk based on ovarian markers. These studies collectively underscore the importance of personalized treatment plans in enhancing the safety and success of ART [13]. These case studies illustrate the transformative potential of integrating ovarian markers like AMH and AFC into routine clinical practice. By leveraging these markers, fertility specialists can tailor treatment protocols to individual patient profiles, thereby significantly mitigating the risk of OHSS and improving overall clinical outcomes in assisted reproductive technologies [13].

6.7 Recent Advances

Recent studies have highlighted several advancements in the use of ovarian markers to prevent ovarian hyperstimulation syndrome (OHSS), a serious complication of controlled ovarian stimulation in assisted reproductive technology (ART) [13, 14].

1. *Anti-Müllerian hormone (AMH) and antral follicle count (AFC)*:

    - *AMH* has been validated as a reliable predictor for OHSS risk, with higher levels indicating a greater likelihood of developing the syndrome. A recent study confirmed that AMH levels above 3.36 ng/mL have a sensitivity of 90.5% and specificity of 81.3% for predicting OHSS [14].
    - *AFC*, assessed through ultrasound, is equally predictive. Women with a high AFC are more likely to experience OHSS, making AFC a critical component of risk assessment in ART cycles [14].
2. *Individualized controlled ovarian stimulation (iCOS)*:
    - Tailoring stimulation protocols based on AMH and AFC levels helps minimize the risk of OHSS. By adjusting gonadotropin doses according to these markers, clinicians can better manage ovarian response, reducing the incidence of OHSS [13].
3. *GnRH antagonist protocols and GnRH agonist triggers*:
    - The use of GnRH antagonists has been shown to significantly reduce the risk of OHSS. Additionally, triggering ovulation with GnRH agonists instead of hCG nearly eliminates the risk of OHSS, especially when combined with embryo cryopreservation [13].

4. *Adjunctive therapies*:
   - Medications such as metformin and cabergoline have emerged as effective adjuncts in OHSS prevention. Metformin reduces the ovarian response to stimulation, while cabergoline inhibits VEGF-mediated vascular permeability, both contributing to a lower incidence of OHSS [13].

These recent advances underline the importance of using ovarian markers like AMH and AFC in personalized treatment protocols to prevent OHSS. By incorporating these markers into clinical practice, alongside newer therapeutic strategies, the safety and effectiveness of ART can be significantly enhanced.

6.8 Conclusion

The role of ovarian markers in preventing ovarian hyperstimulation syndrome (OHSS) represents a significant advancement in reproductive medicine. By leveraging markers such as anti-Müllerian hormone (AMH) and antral follicle count (AFC), clinicians can now better predict and mitigate the risks associated with controlled ovarian stimulation. Individualized treatment protocols based on these markers, combined with novel therapeutic strategies like GnRH antagonist protocols, GnRH agonist triggers, and adjunctive medications, offer a more tailored and safer approach to fertility treatments. These advancements not only improve patient outcomes but also enhance the overall safety and efficacy of assisted reproductive technologies (ART). Through this comprehensive exploration, it is evident that the integration of ovarian markers into clinical practice has the potential to transform the management of OHSS, reducing its incidence and severity. As research continues to evolve, the future of fertility treatment looks promising, with the prospect of even more refined and effective strategies on the horizon. This book serves as a testament to the progress made and a guide for future endeavors in the quest to ensure safer reproductive health care.

References

1. Smith V, Osianlis T, Vollenhoven B. Prevention of ovarian hyperstimulation syndrome: a review. Obstet Gynecol Int. 2015;2015:514159.
2. Practice Committee of the American Society for Reproductive Medicine. Electronic address: asrm@asrm.org. Prevention of moderate and severe ovarian hyperstimulation syndrome: a guideline. Fertil Steril. 2024;121(2):230–45.
3. Devroey P, Polyzos NP, Blockeel C. An OHSS-free clinic by segmentation of IVF treatment. Hum Reprod. 2011;26(10):2593–7.
4. Fiedler K, Ezcurra D. Predicting and preventing ovarian hyperstimulation syndrome (OHSS): the need for individualized not standardized treatment. Reprod Biol Endocrinol. 2012;10:32.
5. Barbosa MAP, Teixeira DM, Navarro PAAS, Ferriani RA, Nastri CO, Martins WP. Impact of endometriosis and its staging on assisted reproduction outcome: systematic review and meta-analysis. Ultrasound Obstet Gynecol. 2014;44(3):261–78.
6. Humaidan P, Quartarolo J, Papanikolaou EG. Preventing ovarian hyperstimulation syndrome: guidance for the clinician. Fertil Steril. 2010;94(2):389–400.
7. Alvarez C, Martí-Bonmatí L, Novella-Maestre E, Sanz R, Gómez R, Fernández-Sánchez M, et al. Dopamine agonist cabergoline reduces hemoconcentration and ascites in hyperstimulated women undergoing assisted reproduction. J Clin Endocrinol Metab. 2007;92(8):2931–7.
8. Tang T, Glanville J, Orsi N, Barth JH, Balen AH. The use of metformin for women with PCOS undergoing IVF treatment. Hum Reprod. 2006;21(6):1416–25.
9. Aboulghar M. Symposium: update on prediction and management of OHSS. Prevent OHSS Reprod Biomed Online. 2009;19(1):33–42.
10. Guo J-L, Zhang D-D, Zhao Y, Zhang D, Zhang X-M, Zhou C-Q, et al. Pharmacologic interventions in preventing ovarian Hyperstimulation syndrome: a systematic review and network meta-analysis. Sci Rep. 2016;6:19093.
11. Delvigne A, Rozenberg S. Epidemiology and prevention of ovarian hyperstimulation syndrome (OHSS): a review. Hum Reprod Update. 2002;8(6):559–77.
12. Rotshenker-Olshinka K, Badeghiesh A, Volodarsky-Perel A, Steiner N, Suarthana E, Dahan MH. Trends in ovarian hyperstimulation syndrome hospitalization rates in the USA: an ongoing concern. Reprod Biomed Online. 2020;41(3):357–60.

13. Palomba S, Costanzi F, Nelson SM, Caserta D, Humaidan P. Interventions to prevent or reduce the incidence and severity of ovarian hyperstimulation syndrome: a systematic umbrella review of the best clinical evidence. Reprod Biol Endocrinol. 2023;21(1):67.
14. Practice Committee of the American Society for Reproductive Medicine. Electronic address: ASRM@asrm.org. Prevention and treatment of moderate and severe ovarian hyperstimulation syndrome: a guideline. Fertil Steril. 2016;106(7):1634–47.

Can Newer Biochemical Markers Prevent OHSS?

7

Sima Simcha Nagawkar Perlov,
Ella Khairish Ben Zeev, and Yuval Or

7.1 Introduction

Ovarian hyperstimulation syndrome (OHSS) is a rare but serious complication arising from controlled ovarian stimulation during fertility treatments. Severe OHSS can lead to life-threatening complications, including acute respiratory distress syndrome (ARDS), pleural effusion, acute renal insufficiency, venous thromboembolism, and even death. Historically, moderate-to-severe OHSS has been reported to occur in approximately 1–5% of in vitro fertilization (IVF) cycles [1–5]. However, accurately estimating its true incidence is challenging due to a lack of consensus on definitions and underreporting in the literature.

OHSS is classified based on the timing of onset as either early or late. Early-onset OHSS occurs after controlled ovarian hyperstimulation and an ovulatory dose of human chorionic gonadotropin (hCG), with symptoms typically arising 4–7 days after the hCG trigger and usually resolving with menses. Late-onset OHSS, in contrast, typically begins at least 9 days after the hCG trigger in

S. S. Nagawkar Perlov (✉) · E. Khairish Ben Zeev · Y. Or
IVF and Fertility Unit, Department of Obstetrics and Gynecology, Kaplan Medical Center, affiliated to the Faculty of Medicine, Hebrew University of Jerusalem, Rehovot, Israel
e-mail: simana1@clalit.org.il; Yuval_O@clalit.org.il

G. N. Allahbadia et al. (eds.), *Ovarian Hyperstimulation Syndrome (OHSS) Free Clinic*, https://doi.org/10.1007/978-981-95-3289-6_7

response to the rising hCG during pregnancy, often presenting more severely and prolonging the course of the condition [6]. Additionally, OHSS is staged according to symptom severity and laboratory findings, categorized as mild, moderate, severe, or critical [7, 8].

Prevention strategies for OHSS can be broadly categorized into primary or secondary approaches. Primary prevention involves classifying patients based on clinical risk factors—such as age, body mass index (BMI), polycystic ovary syndrome (PCOS), and history of previous OHSS—as well as laboratory and sonographic parameters like anti-Müllerian hormone (AMH) levels and antral follicular count (AFC). For at-risk patients, individualized treatment protocols, especially using antagonist protocols, are implemented. Other strategies may include targeting unifollicular ovulation in nonassisted reproductive technology (ART) cycles (reducing gonadotropin doses, using adjunctive therapies like metformin, and using aromatase inhibitors for ovulation induction), individualizing IVF treatment regimens, avoiding hCG for luteal phase support, and considering alternative ovulation triggers [9, 10].

Secondary prevention focuses on managing patients who exhibit excessive responses during a cycle—characterized by elevated serum estradiol (E2), a large number of growing follicles, and a high number of oocytes retrieved—aiming to prevent progression to OHSS. Strategies may include coasting, freezing all embryos or oocytes, and cycle cancellation. Other risk-reducing treatments suggested include colloid or albumin infusion, hydroxyethyl starch (HES), and cabergoline [9, 10].

Tertiary prevention aims to reduce the severity of OHSS and prevent further morbidity. Clinical management depends on the severity of OHSS, the presence of any complications, and whether pregnancy is present. Treatment is primarily supportive, addressing issues such as electrolyte imbalances, hemodynamic changes, liver dysfunction, pulmonary manifestations, hypoglobulinemia, febrile morbidity, thromboembolic events, adnexal torsion or tear, and neurological manifestations [11, 12]. In severe cases where stabilization efforts fail, termination of pregnancy may be necessary.

7.2 Rationale

Preventing OHSS is an important strategy for reducing its incidence. The initial step in this process should be the identification of at-risk patients prior to initiation of ovarian stimulation. Stimulation protocols should be tailored to minimize OHSS risk based on the patient's individual risk profile. While consideration of all risk factors and preventive measures has been shown to decrease both the probability and severity of OHSS, these measures do not eliminate the risk entirely. Consequently, there is a need for more reliable tools to assess this risk. Recent studies highlight new biochemical markers as potential targets for improved evaluation and prevention, which will be discussed further in this chapter.

7.3 Clinical Discussion

Exploring new biochemical markers for identifying and preventing OHSS will be more feasible with a comprehensive understanding of its pathophysiology. A significant barrier to proactive measures is the unclear molecular etiology of OHSS. Current knowledge indicates that the hallmark of OHSS is increased capillary permeability, leading to fluid shifts from the intravascular space to extravascular compartments [13, 14]. Vascular endothelial growth factor (VEGF) plays a crucial role in this process by enhancing vascular permeability [15]. Other factors, including angiotensin II, insulin-like growth factor, epidermal growth factor, transforming growth factors (alpha and beta), basic fibroblast growth factor, platelet-derived growth factor, interleukin-1B, and interleukin-6, may also contribute to the development and severity of OHSS [16]. Additionally, the intraovarian renin-angiotensin system (RAS) is implicated in the condition [17, 18]. A more detailed discussion of OHSS pathophysiology can be found in a separate chapter.

Some ovarian biomarkers have been extensively studied and are currently utilized in clinical practice. For instance, measuring

AMH levels helps identify patients at risk, allowing adjustments in treatment protocols. Elevated E2 levels during treatment indicate cases where ovulation triggering with hCG should be avoided, thereby minimizing the occurrence and severity of OHSS. VEGF, secreted by granulosa cells and stimulated by hCG, is another vital biomarker, as mentioned earlier. Research shows that higher VEGF levels correlate with increased severity of OHSS [16]. Consequently, VEGF has been targeted by various drugs aimed at blocking its function, with cabergoline being the most commonly used due to its anti-VEGF activity. It has demonstrated effectiveness and safety in preventing severe OHSS [16]. A detailed discussion of these biomarkers and their clinical applications is provided in another chapter.

Numerous studies have explored other proteins potentially involved in the pathophysiology of OHSS, which may serve as additional treatment targets alongside VEGF. The human follicular fluid offers a significant microenvironment for maintaining the physiological functions of the ovarian follicle. Collecting this fluid during oocyte retrieval enables its use for research and for identifying biochemical markers relevant to the prediction, diagnosis, and treatment of OHSS. Research indicates that the content and concentration of certain proteins and biochemical markers differ between OHSS and non-OHSS patients. This chapter will briefly summarize recent biomarker research aimed at identifying those associated with severe OHSS, which could lead to potential prevention strategies. We will focus on markers primarily studied in humans, avoiding animal model discussions, and will not delve into specific biological methods or molecular signaling pathways to keep the focus on clinical practice.

7.3.1 Transforming Growth Factor-Beta (TGF-β)

The TGF-β superfamily includes TGF-βs, activins/inhibins, AMH, bone morphogenetic proteins (BMPs), growth differentiation factors (GDFs), and other proteins that regulate various physiological and pathological events in the ovary [19]. Immunohistochemical analyses reveal that TGF-β1 protein is expressed in both human granulosa and theca cells [20, 21]. Certain cytokines and growth factors, including TGF-β1, can elevate VEGF levels and induce its secretion in different cell types [22]. It was demonstrated that TGF-β1 stimulates VEGF expression and secretion from human granulosa-lutein (hGL) cells through various signaling pathways. Notably, TGF-β1 and VEGF levels in follicular fluid were positively correlated and significantly increased in OHSS patients compared to controls [23]. Another study highlighted that TGF-β3 is also present in follicular fluid and is elevated in OHSS patients [24]. These findings enhance our understanding of the mechanisms mediating VEGF expression in hGL cells and suggest that targeting TGF-β1 and TGF-β3 signaling may offer alternative strategies for preventing OHSS.

7.3.2 Secreted Protein Acidic and Rich in Cysteine (SPARC)

SPARC, also known as osteonectin or BM-40, is a multifunctional matricellular glycoprotein secreted by various cell types. Earlier studies have reported its expression in human ovaries, with mRNA levels of SPARC decreasing in postmenopausal ovaries [25]. Additionally, SPARC expression is downregulated in granulosa cells from PCOS patients with insulin resistance compared to normal controls [26]. Recent findings indicate that SPARC protein levels in follicular fluid are higher in OHSS patients than in those without the condition [27]. Furthermore, TGF-β1 treatment upregulates SPARC protein expression in hGL cells, and SPARC is involved in the TGF-β1-induced expression of VEGF and aromatase [27]. These results reveal a novel regulatory mechanism for SPARC in hGL cells, enhancing our understanding of its physiological and pathological roles in the ovary, which could imply therapeutic approaches for OHSS.

7.3.3 Growth Differentiation Factor-8 (GDF-8)

GDF-8, or myostatin, is a member of the TGF-β superfamily, primarily synthesized by skeletal muscle cells. Its activity is regulated by various factors, and it influences adipogenesis beyond the musculoskeletal system; aberrant GDF-8 expression is linked to obesity [28]. Emerging evidence suggests that GDF-8 plays a role in female reproductive functions, with its expression and receptors detected in the ovary, uterus, and placenta [29–31]. GDF-8 and its receptors are expressed in human granulosa cells, and secreted GDF-8 has been found in ovarian follicular fluid [31–34]. Levels of GDF-8 are elevated in the follicular fluid of OHSS patients compared to controls, and pretreatment with GDF-8 increases aromatase expression in hGL cells [35]. This suggests that GDF-8 may stimulate aromatase expression and E2 production in granulosa cells, contributing to the pathogenesis of OHSS. Understanding these mechanisms may lead to alternative therapeutic strategies and the use of GDF-8 signaling pathways as potential markers for OHSS prevention.

7.3.4 Epidermal Growth Factor Receptor (EGFR) and Amphiregulin (AREG)

EGFR, also known as HER1/ErbB1 and HER2 (ErbB2), belongs to a family of receptor tyrosine kinases that regulate various physiological and pathological events [36]. In reproductive tissues, EGFR and its ligands mediate several female reproductive functions [37]. In the ovary, EGFR and its coreceptor HER2 are expressed in granulosa cells [38, 39]. Among the ligands, AREG is the most abundant in human follicular fluid [40]. Transcripts for AREG, EGFR, and HER2 are elevated in granulosa cells, and AREG protein levels in the follicular fluid of OHSS patients are significantly higher. A positive correlation exists between follicular fluid AREG protein levels and various OHSS indices, including VEGF levels in granulosa cells. AREG treatment has been shown to enhance VEGF expression in granulosa cells of OHSS patients more rapidly than in controls. Moreover, knocking down EGFR and AREG attenuates the stimulatory effect of hCG on VEGF [41]. These findings underscore AREG's crucial role in OHSS development and suggest that targeting EGFR/HER2-mediated signaling may offer novel prevention and treatment strategies.

7.3.5 Melatonin

During OHSS pathogenesis, excessive production of angiotensin II, VEGF, interleukins, nitric oxide, and tumor necrosis factor-alpha contributes to an imbalance between reactive oxygen species (ROS) and antioxidants [42]. This oxidative stress compromises the vascular endothelium, leading to heightened permeability and exacerbating OHSS [43]. Melatonin, primarily secreted by the pineal gland, is regulated by circadian rhythms, but its levels are higher in follicular fluid than in plasma, as it is also synthesized in the ovary, primarily by granulosa cells [44]. Melatonin and its metabolites are potent radical scavengers, reducing ROS levels in the ovary through various mechanisms, thus protecting oocytes and granulosa cells from oxidative damage [45, 46].

Sestrins, stress-inducible metabolic regulators, are widely expressed in adult tissues [47, 48]. Sestrin-2 (SESN2) acts as a suppressor of ROS accumulation and protects neurons [49]. Overexpression of SESN2 decreases ROS levels, while its knockdown increases ROS content [50, 51]. A recent study found significantly higher SESN2 levels in high-risk OHSS patients compared to controls, likely due to increased oxidative stress. Additionally, SESN2 levels were positively correlated with ROS generation in cultured human granulosa cells. Treatment with melatonin significantly reduced SESN2 levels and ROS, thereby decreasing cell apoptosis [52]. These findings suggest that melatonin could be a promising therapeutic agent for the treatment and prevention of OHSS.

7.3.6 Coagulation and Fibrinolysis Biomarkers

Women with OHSS exhibit increased vascular permeability, leading to fluid shifts that can result in a hypercoagulable state and potential thrombosis. Currently, no single blood test reliably reflects changes in the early stages of OHSS. However, sensitive biomarkers in the hemostatic system, such as the thrombin-antithrombin complex (TAT), plasmin alpha2-plasmin inhibitor complex (PIC), soluble thrombomodulin (sTM), and tissue plasminogen activator-inhibitor complex (TPAI-C), may indicate even minimal hemostatic activation [53]. Studies show significantly higher levels of TAT, PIC, and TPAI-C, along with lower sTM levels, in OHSS patients compared to controls. Furthermore, TAT, PIC, and TPAI-C levels were notably elevated in patients with severe OHSS compared to those with mild to moderate cases. These findings can help establish cutoff levels for different severity stages [54]. Since these biomarkers can be quickly and easily measured through blood tests, they may assist in early detection of severe OHSS and help identify high-risk patients requiring closer monitoring and potential early prophylactic anticoagulation therapy.

7.3.7 Lipid Analysis of Follicular Fluid

Dyslipidemia may contribute to OHSS development, suggesting that abnormal lipid metabolism could be a risk factor [55]. Proteomic analyses have indicated that lipoprotein lipase may serve as a predictive marker for OHSS in PCOS patients [56, 57]. Therefore, it is reasonable to hypothesize a strong relationship between lipid metabolism and OHSS occurrence. The lipid content in follicular fluid is relatively stable compared to blood samples, making lipidomic analysis of follicular fluid a valuable approach for identifying potential biomarkers for OHSS [58]. Recent study has shown significant differences in lipid profiles between OHSS patients and controls, with higher levels of cholesterol ester (ChE) observed in the OHSS group, indicating its potential as a future biomarker [59].

7.4 Recent Advance

To date, prevention strategies for OHSS have primarily focused on identifying at-risk patients based on clinical, sonographic, and laboratory factors. This information allows for tailored adjustments to treatment protocols prior to or during assisted reproductive technology (ART) based on individual responses to ovarian stimulation. Recent research has highlighted biochemical markers that play a critical role in the pathophysiology of OHSS, suggesting that these markers could serve as potential targets for prevention and treatment, as well as for reducing severity. However, their efficacy has only been studied in laboratory settings and has yet to be tested in clinical trials or with specific commercial drugs. Further research is essential to establish their clinical applicability for routine use.

In addition to biochemical markers, innovative approaches such as DNA genotyping and RNA sequencing may help identify genes involved in OHSS pathophysiology [42, 60–62]. In the future, it may be possible to identify women at high risk for developing OHSS using simple genetic tools that reveal gene variations associated with increased risk.

7.5 Conclusion

Biochemical markers have the potential to serve as targets for preventing the occurrence of OHSS, reducing its severity, or guiding treatment strategies. However, current data are largely theoretical, and no validated clinical marker has emerged as superior to others. Additionally, no specific commercial drug has been developed or tested for this purpose. As a result, strong evidence-based support for widespread routine clinical use remains lacking, with these markers primarily applicable in research contexts. Further clinical research is essential to establish their role in clinical practice.

References

1. Steward RG, Lan L, Shah AA, Yeh JS, Price TM, Goldfarb JM, et al. Oocyte number as a predictor for ovarian hyperstimulation syndrome and live birth: an analysis of 256,381 in vitro fertilization cycles. Fertil Steril. 2014;101(4):967–73.
2. Luke B, Brown MB, Morbeck DE, Hudson SB, Coddington CC, Stern JE. Factors associated with ovarian hyperstimulation syndrome (OHSS) and its effect on assisted reproductive technology (ART) treatment and outcome. Fertil Steril. 2010;94(4):1399–404.
3. Jayaprakasan K, Chan Y, Islam R, Haoula Z, Hopkisson J, Coomarasamy A, et al. Prediction of in vitro fertilization outcome at different antral follicle count thresholds in a prospective cohort of 1,012 women. Fertil Steril. 2012;98(3):657–63.
4. Kahnberg A, Enskog A, Brännström M, Lundin K, Bergh C. Prediction of ovarian hyperstimulation syndrome in women undergoing in vitro fertilization. Acta Obstet Gynecol Scand. 2009;88(12):1373–81.
5. Papanikolaou EG, Pozzobon C, Kolibianakis EM, Camus M, Tournaye H, Fatemi HM, et al. Incidence and prediction of ovarian hyperstimulation syndrome in women undergoing gonadotropin-releasing hormone antagonist in vitro fertilization cycles. Fertil Steril. 2006;85(1):112–20.
6. Mathur RS, Akande AV, Keay SD, Hunt LP, Jenkins JM. Distinction between early and late ovarian hyperstimulation syndrome. Fertil Steril. 2000;73(5):901–7.
7. Navot D, Bergh PA, Laufer N. Ovarian hyperstimulation syndrome in novel reproductive technologies: prevention and treatment. Fertil Steril. 1992;58(2):249–61.
8. Fiedler K, Ezcurra D. Predicting and preventing ovarian hyperstimulation syndrome (OHSS): the need for individualized not standardized treatment. Reprod Biol Endocrinol. 2012;10:32.
9. Smith V, Osianlis T, Vollenhoven B. Prevention of ovarian hyperstimulation syndrome: a review. Obstet Gynecol Int. 2015;2015:514159.
10. Practice Committee of the American Society for Reproductive Medicine. Electronic address: asrm@asrm.org. Prevention of moderate and severe ovarian hyperstimulation syndrome: a guideline. Fertil Steril. 2024;121(2):230–45.
11. Delvigne A, Rozenberg S. Review of clinical course and treatment of ovarian hyperstimulation syndrome (OHSS). Hum Reprod Update. 2003;9(1):77–96.

12. Brinsden PR, Wada I, Tan SL, Balen A, Jacobs HS. Diagnosis, prevention and management of ovarian hyperstimulation syndrome. Br J Obstet Gynaecol. 1995;102(10):767–72.
13. Goldsman MP, Pedram A, Dominguez CE, Ciuffardi I, Levin E, Asch RH. Increased capillary permeability induced by human follicular fluid: a hypothesis for an ovarian origin of the hyperstimulation syndrome. Fertil Steril. 1995;63(2):268–72.
14. Tollan A, Holst N, Forsdahl F, Fadnes HO, Oian P, Maltau JM. Transcapillary fluid dynamics during ovarian stimulation for in vitro fertilization. Am J Obstet Gynecol. 1990;162(2):554–8.
15. Pellicer A, Albert C, Mercader A, Bonilla-Musoles F, Remohí J, Simón C. The pathogenesis of ovarian hyperstimulation syndrome: in vivo studies investigating the role of interleukin-1beta, interleukin-6, and vascular endothelial growth factor. Fertil Steril. 1999;71(3):482–9.
16. Naredi N, Talwar P, Sandeep K. VEGF antagonist for the prevention of ovarian hyperstimulation syndrome: current status. Med J Armed Forces India. 2014;70(1):58–63.
17. Herr D, Bekes I, Wulff C. Local renin-angiotensin system in the reproductive system. Front Endocrinol (Lausanne). 2013;4:150.
18. Schwentner L, Wöckel A, Herr D, Wulff C. Is there a role of the local tissue RAS in the regulation of physiologic and pathophysiologic conditions in the reproductive tract? J Renin-Angiotensin-Aldosterone Syst. 2011;12(4):385–93.
19. Knight PG, Glister C. TGF-beta superfamily members and ovarian follicle development. Reproduction. 2006;132(2):191–206.
20. Chegini N, Flanders KC. Presence of transforming growth factor-beta and their selective cellular localization in human ovarian tissue of various reproductive stages. Endocrinology. 1992;130(3):1707–15.
21. Chegini N, Williams RS. Immunocytochemical localization of transforming growth factors (TGFs) TGF-alpha and TGF-beta in human ovarian tissues. J Clin Endocrinol Metab. 1992;74(5):973–80.
22. Ferrara N, Davis-Smyth T. The biology of vascular endothelial growth factor. Endocr Rev. 1997;18(1):4–25.
23. Liu B, Jia Q, Hong I-S, Dang X, Wu Z, Wang H, et al. TGF-β1 and TGF-β3, but not TGF-β2, are upregulated in the ovaries of ovarian hyperstimulation syndrome†. Biol Reprod. 2024;110(1):116–29.
24. Fang L, Li Y, Wang S, Li Y, Chang H-M, Yi Y, et al. TGF-β1 induces VEGF expression in human granulosa-lutein cells: a potential mechanism for the pathogenesis of ovarian hyperstimulation syndrome. Exp Mol Med. 2020;52(3):450–60.
25. Oksjoki S, Rahkonen O, Haarala M, Vuorio E, Anttila L. Differences in connective tissue gene expression between normally functioning, polycystic and post-menopausal ovaries. Mol Hum Reprod. 2004;10(1):7–14.
26. Kaur S, Archer KJ, Devi MG, Kriplani A, Strauss JF, Singh R. Differential gene expression in granulosa cells from polycystic ovary syndrome

patients with and without insulin resistance: identification of susceptibility gene sets through network analysis. J Clin Endocrinol Metab. 2012;97(10):E2016–21.
27. Dang X, Fang L, Jia Q, Wu Z, Guo Y, Liu B, et al. TGF-β1 upregulates secreted protein acidic and rich in cysteine expression in human granulosa-lutein cells: a potential mechanism for the pathogenesis of ovarian hyperstimulation syndrome. Cell Commun Signal. 2023;21(1):101.
28. Zamani N, Brown CW. Emerging roles for the transforming growth factor-{beta} superfamily in regulating adiposity and energy expenditure. Endocr Rev. 2011;32(3):387–403.
29. Islam MS, Catherino WH, Protic O, Janjusevic M, Gray PC, Giannubilo SR, et al. Role of activin-a and myostatin and their signaling pathway in human myometrial and leiomyoma cell function. J Clin Endocrinol Metab. 2014;99(5):E775–85.
30. Peiris HN, Salomon C, Payton D, Ashman K, Vaswani K, Chan A, et al. Myostatin is localized in extravillous trophoblast and up-regulates migration. J Clin Endocrinol Metab. 2014;99(11):E2288–97.
31. Lin T-T, Chang H-M, Hu X-L, Leung PCK, Zhu Y-M. Follicular localization of growth differentiation factor 8 and its receptors in normal and polycystic ovary syndrome ovaries. Biol Reprod. 2018;98(5):683–94.
32. Chang H-M, Fang L, Cheng J-C, Klausen C, Sun Y-P, Leung PCK. Growth differentiation factor 8 down-regulates pentraxin 3 in human granulosa cells. Mol Cell Endocrinol. 2015;404:82–90.
33. Fang L, Yu Y, Zhang R, He J, Sun Y-P. Serum GDF-8 levels change dynamically during controlled ovarian hyperstimulation in patients undergoing IVF/ICSI-ET. Sci Rep. 2016;6:28036.
34. Fang L, Wang S, Li Y, Yu Y, Li Y, Yan Y, et al. High GDF-8 in follicular fluid is associated with a low pregnancy rate in IVF patients with PCOS. Reproduction. 2020;160(1):11–9.
35. Fang L, Yan Y, Wang S, Guo Y, Li Y, Jia Q, et al. High ovarian GDF-8 levels contribute to elevated estradiol production in ovarian hyperstimulation syndrome by stimulating aromatase expression. Int J Biol Sci. 2021;17(9):2338–47.
36. Hynes NE, MacDonald G. ErbB receptors and signaling pathways in cancer. Curr Opin Cell Biol. 2009;21(2):177–84.
37. Schneider MR, Wolf E. The epidermal growth factor receptor and its ligands in female reproduction: insights from rodent models. Cytokine Growth Factor Rev. 2008;19(2):173–81.
38. Noma N, Kawashima I, Fan H-Y, Fujita Y, Kawai T, Tomoda Y, et al. LH-induced neuregulin 1 (NRG1) type III transcripts control granulosa cell differentiation and oocyte maturation. Mol Endocrinol. 2011;25(1):104–16.
39. Maruo T, Ladines-Llave CA, Samoto T, Matsuo H, Manalo AS, Ito H, et al. Expression of epidermal growth factor and its receptor in the human

ovary during follicular growth and regression. Endocrinology. 1993;132(2):924–31.

40. Zamah AM, Hsieh M, Chen J, Vigne JL, Rosen MP, Cedars MI, et al. Human oocyte maturation is dependent on LH-stimulated accumulation of the epidermal growth factor-like growth factor, amphiregulin. Hum Reprod. 2010;25(10):2569–78.
41. Fang L, Yu Y, Li Y, Wang S, He J, Zhang R, et al. Up-regulation of AREG, EGFR and HER2 contributes to increased VEGF expression in granulosa cells of patients with OHSS†. Biol Reprod. 2019;
42. Daghestani MH, Alqahtani HA, AlBakheet A, Al Deery M, Awartani KA, Daghestani MH, et al. Global transcriptional profiling of granulosa cells from polycystic ovary syndrome patients: comparative analyses of patients with or without history of ovarian Hyperstimulation syndrome reveals distinct biomarkers and pathways. J Clin Med. 2022;11(23)
43. Gómez R, Soares SR, Busso C, Garcia-Velasco JA, Simón C, Pellicer A. Physiology and pathology of ovarian hyperstimulation syndrome. Semin Reprod Med. 2010;28(6):448–57.
44. Brzezinski A, Seibel MM, Lynch HJ, Deng MH, Wurtman RJ. Melatonin in human preovulatory follicular fluid. J Clin Endocrinol Metab. 1987;64(4):865–7.
45. Zavodnik IB, Domanski AV, Lapshina EA, Bryszewska M, Reiter RJ. Melatonin directly scavenges free radicals generated in red blood cells and a cell-free system: chemiluminescence measurements and theoretical calculations. Life Sci. 2006;79(4):391–400.
46. Kang J-T, Koo O-J, Kwon D-K, Park H-J, Jang G, Kang S-K, et al. Effects of melatonin on in vitro maturation of porcine oocyte and expression of melatonin receptor RNA in cumulus and granulosa cells. J Pineal Res. 2009;46(1):22–8.
47. Velasco-Miguel S, Buckbinder L, Jean P, Gelbert L, Talbott R, Laidlaw J, et al. PA26, a novel target of the p53 tumor suppressor and member of the GADD family of DNA damage and growth arrest inducible genes. Oncogene. 1999;18(1):127–37.
48. Querfurth HW, LaFerla FM. Alzheimer's disease. N Engl J Med. 2010;362(4):329–44.
49. Wullschleger S, Loewith R, Hall MN. TOR signaling in growth and metabolism. Cell. 2006;124(3):471–84.
50. Budanov AV, Sablina AA, Feinstein E, Koonin EV, Chumakov PM. Regeneration of peroxiredoxins by p53-regulated sestrins, homologs of bacterial AhpD. Science. 2004;304(5670):596–600.
51. Kopnin PB, Agapova LS, Kopnin BP, Chumakov PM. Repression of sestrin family genes contributes to oncogenic Ras-induced reactive oxygen species up-regulation and genetic instability. Cancer Res. 2007;67(10):4671–8.

52. Zheng M, Liu M, Zhang C. Melatonin ameliorates ovarian Hyperstimulation syndrome (OHSS) through SESN2 regulated Antiapoptosis. Obstet Gynecol Int. 2023;2023:1121227.
53. Mei H, Jiang Y, Luo L, Huang R, Su L, Hou M, et al. Evaluation the combined diagnostic value of TAT, PIC, tPAIC, and sTM in disseminated intravascular coagulation: a multi-center prospective observational study. Thromb Res. 2019;173:20–6.
54. Li S, Qian Y, Pei Y, Wu K, Lu S. Coagulation and fibrinolysis biomarkers as potential indicators for the diagnosis and classification of ovarian hyperstimulation syndrome. Front Med (Lausanne). 2021;8:720342.
55. Liu F, Jiang Q, Sun X, Huang Y, Zhang Z, Han T, et al. Lipid metabolic disorders and ovarian hyperstimulation syndrome: a retrospective analysis. Front Physiol. 2020;11:491892.
56. Wu L, Sun Y, Wan J, Luan T, Cheng Q, Tan Y. A proteomic analysis identifies candidate early biomarkers to predict ovarian hyperstimulation syndrome in polycystic ovarian syndrome patients. Mol Med Report. 2017;16(1):272–80.
57. Mead JR, Irvine SA, Ramji DP. Lipoprotein lipase: structure, function, regulation, and role in disease. J Mol Med. 2002;80(12):753–69.
58. Cordeiro FB, Cataldi TR, Perkel KJ, et al. Lipidomics analysis of follicular fluid by ESI-MS reveals potential biomarkers for ovarian endometriosis. J Assist Reprod Genet. 2015;32(12):1817–25.
59. Gao Y, Li J, Fan S, Chen P, Huang M, Bi H. Lipid analysis of follicular fluids by UHPLC-ESI-HRMS discovers potential biomarkers for ovarian Hyperstimulation syndrome. Front Endocrinol (Lausanne). 2022;13:895116.
60. Yan B, Wu B, Wang Z-Q, Wei Y, Ni Y-L. Peripheral blood transcriptome analysis of patients with ovarian hyperstimulation syndrome through high-throughput sequencing. Reprod Dev Med. 2023;7(2):115–21.
61. Zhao C, Liu X, Shi Z, Zhang J, Zhang J, Jia X, et al. Role of serum miRNAs in the prediction of ovarian hyperstimulation syndrome in polycystic ovarian syndrome patients. Cell Physiol Biochem. 2015;35(3):1086–94.
62. O'Brien TJ, Harralson AF, Tran T, Gindoff I, Orkunoglu-Suer FE, Frankfurter D, et al. Kinase insert domain receptor/vascular endothelial growth factor receptor 2 (KDR) genetic variation is associated with ovarian hyperstimulation syndrome. Reprod Biol Endocrinol. 2014;12:36.

The Role of Ultrasound in the Prevention and Prediction of Ovarian Hyperstimulation Syndrome

8

Miremberg Hadas,
Krajden Haratz Karina, and Wolman Igal

8.1 Introduction

Ovarian hyperstimulation syndrome (OHSS) is a potentially serious complication associated with ovarian stimulation in assisted reproductive technology (ART) cycles [1]. The ability to predict and prevent OHSS is crucial for optimizing patient outcomes in fertility treatments. Ultrasound plays a pivotal role in addressing those issues.

This chapter will explore the various ultrasound-based strategies utilized in identifying patients at risk of OHSS and implementing preventive measures to mitigate its occurrence.

Identifying Women at Risk Before Commencing Ovarian Stimulation.

Women predisposed to a high ovarian response can be identified prior to ovarian stimulation (OS) through various indicators.

M. Hadas · K. H. Karina · W. Igal (✉)
Ultrasound Unit in Obstetrics and Gynecology, Lis Maternity Hospital, Tel-Aviv Medical, Tel Aviv, Israel
e-mail: hadasmi@tlvmc.gov.il; karinakra@tlvmc.gov.il

G. N. Allahbadia et al. (eds.), *Ovarian Hyperstimulation Syndrome (OHSS) Free Clinic*, https://doi.org/10.1007/978-981-95-3289-6_8

These include ovarian reserve markers such as anti-Müllerian hormone (AMH) and antral follicle count (AFC). Other factors include age, previous history of high response to OS, ovarian morphology, FSH receptor polymorphisms, and body mass index (BMI). In this chapter, we will focus on ultrasound parameters.

Ultrasound parameters.

- *Ovarian morphology.*

Polycystic ovaries (Fig. 8.1) exhibit increased sensitivity to gonadotropin stimulation in comparison to normal ovaries. This heightened sensitivity leads to the development of a greater number of pre-antral follicles that are responsive to ovarian stimulation [2].

- *Ovarian vascularity.*

Transvaginal pulsed Doppler has been widely utilized to evaluate ovarian blood flow patterns in both natural and stimulated cycles [3]. Ovarian blood vessel resistance tends to be lower in the ovary containing the dominant follicle or corpus luteum in comparison to the opposite ovary [4]. The day of the LH surge typically exhibits the least vascular resistance, whereas the first day of menses shows the highest resistance.

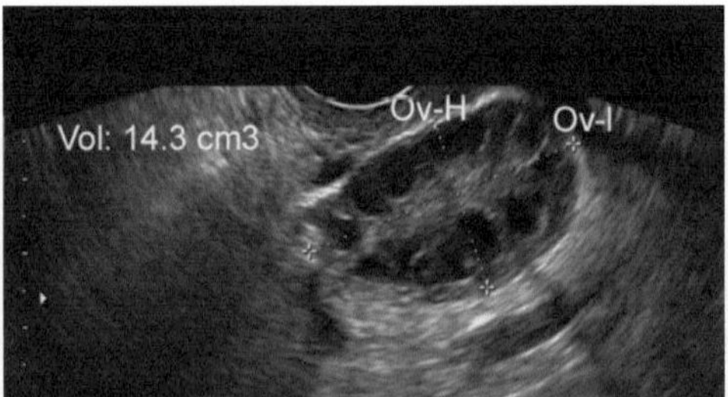

Fig. 8.1 Polycystic ovary

Measuring vascular resistance and flow velocity around developing follicles is feasible. As the follicle diameter expands, vascular resistance diminishes, leading to an increase in flow velocity [5].

Color Doppler imaging of ovarian vascular mapping offers a novel functional approach to identifying OHSS [6] (Fig. 8.2). Local vascular factors promoting ovarian angiogenesis and heightened capillary permeability, triggered by HCG injection, are pivotal in this syndrome [7]. Two distinct patterns of 3D vascular images, observed on days 8–10 of stimulation, correlate with specific serum E2 levels. The "reassuring pattern" exhibits regularly marginally dilated vessels with few coils and a resistive index (RI) of 0.55–0.61, associated with serum E2 levels of 3000–5000 pg/mL, indicating a low risk of OHSS. Conversely, the "aggressive pattern" displays markedly dilated vessels with irregular branching and several coils, along with an RI of 0.48–0.52, and serum E2 levels exceeding 5000–7000 pg/mL, suggesting a higher likelihood of OHSS [8, 9].

- *Antral follicle count (AFC).*

Follicles are oocytes surrounded by granulosa cells that undergo slow early growth characterized by a slight increase in

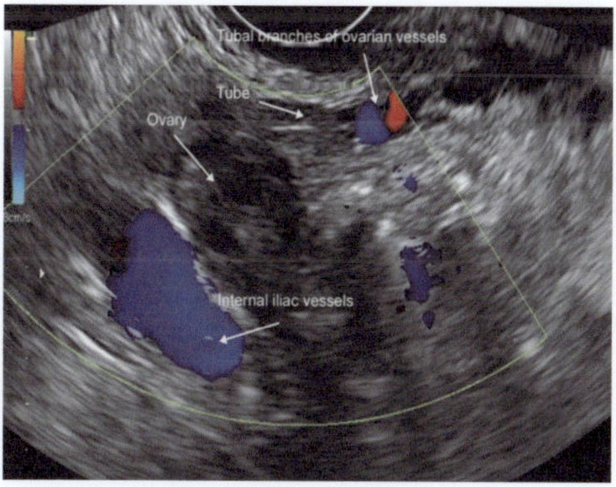

Fig. 8.2 Color Doppler mapping of vasculature

oocyte volume, granulosa cell proliferation, and expansion of the antral cavity. Transitioning to 2-mm pre-antral follicles typically takes about 6 months. The small subset of follicles progressing to the antral stage (> 2 mm) is highly sensitive and responsive to FSH. These follicles, capable of maturing during controlled ovarian stimulation (COS), may serve as predictors for the development of OHSS and a high response to COS. It is advisable to assess AFC between days 2 and 4 of a spontaneous menstrual cycle, in the absence of a follicle >10 mm [10].

Both 2D and 3D ultrasound (US) (Figs. 8.3 and 8.4) can be utilized for assessing antral follicle count (AFC). On 2D US, ovarian follicles are often counted using either real-time or stored

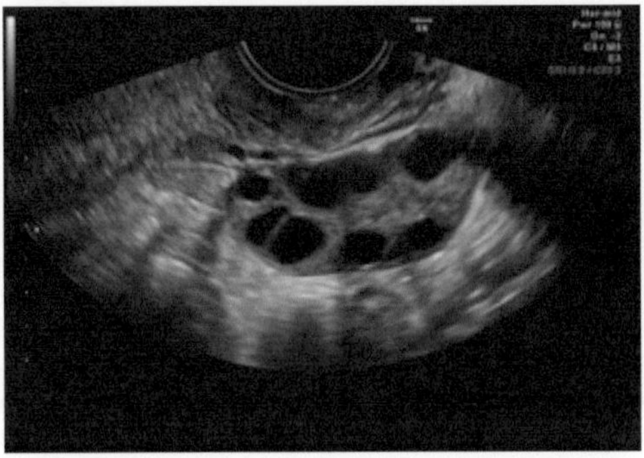

Fig. 8.3 Follicular antral count in 2D

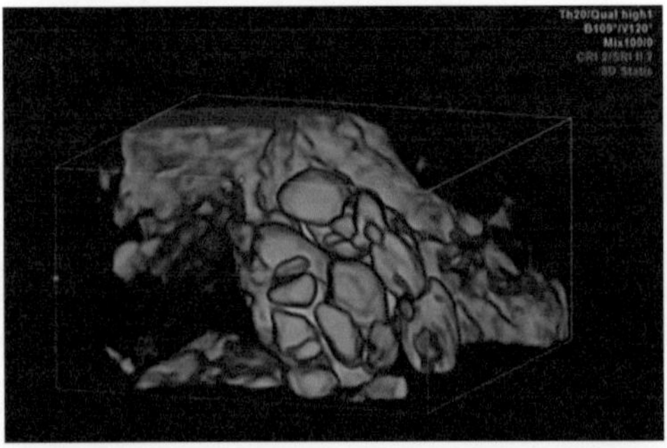

Fig. 8.4 Follicular antral count in 3D

cine loops. In contrast, on 3D US, the follicles are typically manually counted in multiplanar mode. However, counting may also be performed using rendered modes, such as inversion mode, or semiautomatically through sonography-based automated volume calculation [11]. A total AFC ≥ 20 is related to exaggerated ovarian response and a higher risk of OHSS [12].

8.2 Monitoring Ovarian Response During Stimulation

Serial ultrasound examinations are performed during ovarian stimulation to monitor follicular growth and assess ovarian response [13]. Ultrasound allows real-time visualization of developing follicles and enables the adjustment of gonadotropin dosages based on follicular response. Monitoring follicular growth and estradiol levels through ultrasound-guided measurements facilitates the timely identification of patients at risk of excessive ovarian response and OHSS development.

The number of follicles stimulated during COS directly correlates with the level of ovarian stimulation. Evaluating the level of stimulation just before triggering can be done through ultrasound examination by counting the number of medium and large follicles. This assessment parameter can aid in gauging the risk of OHSS and assist in determining the adoption of preventive measures [13, 14].

Various thresholds for defining a high ovarian response have been proposed, and different cutoffs regarding the number of follicles associated with a significantly elevated risk of OHSS have been recommended by different organizations.

According to the guidelines of the European Society of Human Reproduction and Embryology (ESHRE), in a GnRH agonist cycle, an ovarian response of 18 follicles ≥11 mm is deemed to pose an increased risk of OHSS, prompting the recommendation of preventive measures [13]. Conversely, the guidelines of the American Society for Reproductive Medicine (ASRM) identify an exaggerated response to ovarian stimulation as the presence of over 24 follicles (without specifying their size) [15].

Lastly, the International Committee for Monitoring Assisted Reproductive Technologies (ICMART) consensus defines an exaggerated response to ovarian stimulation as the presence of more than 20 follicles measuring over 12 mm [16].

A high response after oocyte pick-up can be confirmed based on the number of oocytes retrieved [13, 15].

Preventing OHSS requires a personalized approach based on individual patient factors and close monitoring throughout the treatment cycle. Individualized gonadotropin dosing based on follicular growth and serum estradiol levels helps minimize the risk of excessive ovarian response [17].

8.3 Conclusion

Ultrasound imaging plays a pivotal role in predicting and preventing ovarian hyperstimulation syndrome in patients undergoing assisted reproductive technology cycles. By enabling the identification of high-risk patients and facilitating individualized stimulation protocols, ultrasound contributes significantly to optimizing patient safety and treatment outcomes in fertility treatments. Continued research and technological advancements in ultrasound imaging hold promise for further improving the prediction and prevention of OHSS in ART cycles.

References

1. Selter J, Wen T, Palmerola KL, Friedman AM, Williams Z, Forman EJ. Life-threatening complications among women with severe ovarian hyperstimulation syndrome. Am J Obstet Gynecol. 2019:220. https://doi.org/10.1016/j.ajog.2019.02.009.
2. Zhu RY, Wong YC, Yong EL. Sonographic evaluation of polycystic ovaries. Best Pract Res Clin Obstet Gynaecol. 2016:37. https://doi.org/10.1016/j.bpobgyn.2016.02.005.
3. Chui DKC, Pugh ND, Walker SM, Gregory L, Shaw RW. Follicular vascularity-the predictive value of transvaginal power Doppler ultrasonography in an in-vitro fertilization programme: a preliminary study. Hum Reprod. 1997:12. https://doi.org/10.1093/humrep/12.1.191.

4. Collins W, Jurkovic D, Bourne T, Kurjak A, Campbell S. Ovarian morphology, endocrine function and intra-follicular blood flow during the peri-ovulatory period. Hum Reprod. 1991:6. https://doi.org/10.1093/oxfordjournals.humrep.a137332.
5. Balakier H, Stronell RD. Color Doppler assessment of folliculogenesis in in vitro fertilization patients. Fertil Steril. 1994:62. https://doi.org/10.1016/s0015-0282(16)57187-8.
6. Shrestha SM, Costello MF, Sjoblom P, McNally G, Bennett M, Steigrad SJ, et al. Power doppler ultrasound assessment of follicular vascularity in the early follicular phase and its relationship with outcome of in vitro fertilization. J Assist Reprod Genet. 2006:23. https://doi.org/10.1007/s10815-006-9029-1.
7. Moohan JM, Healy D, Curcio K, Hurley V, Leoni M. Low intraovarian vascular resistance: a marker for severe ovarian hyperstimulation syndrome. Fertil Steril. 1997:67. https://doi.org/10.1016/S0015-0282(97)81374-X.
8. Jayaprakasan K, Jayaprakasan R, Al-Hasie HA, Clewes JS, Campbell BK, Johnson IR, et al. Can quantitative three-dimensional power Doppler angiography be used to predict ovarian hyperstimulation syndrome? Ultrasound Obstet Gynecol. 2009:33. https://doi.org/10.1002/uog.6373.
9. Nastri CO, Teixeira DM, Moroni RM, Leitão VMS, Martins WP. Ovarian hyperstimulation syndrome: pathophysiology, staging, prediction and prevention. Ultrasound Obstet Gynecol. 2015:45. https://doi.org/10.1002/uog.14684.
10. Broekmans FJM, De Ziegler D, Howles CM, Gougeon A, Trew G, Olivennes F. The antral follicle count: practical recommendations for better standardization. Fertil Steril. 2010:94. https://doi.org/10.1016/j.fertnstert.2009.04.040.
11. Coelho Neto MA, Ludwin A, Borrell A, Benacerraf B, Dewailly D, da Silva CF, et al. Counting ovarian antral follicles by ultrasound: a practical guide. Ultrasound Obstet Gynecol. 2018:51. https://doi.org/10.1002/uog.18945.
12. Ng EHY, Tang OS, Ho PC. The significance of the number of antral follicles prior to stimulation in predicting ovarian responses in an IVF programme. Hum Reprod. 2000:15. https://doi.org/10.1093/humrep/15.9.1937.
13. Bosch E, Broer S, Griesinger G, Grynberg M, Humaidan P, Kolibianakis E, et al. ESHRE guideline: ovarian stimulation for IVF/ICSI. Hum Reprod Open. 2021;2020 https://doi.org/10.1093/hropen/hoaa009.
14. Broer SL, Dólleman M, Van Disseldorp J, Broeze KA, Opmeer BC, Bossuyt PMM, et al. Prediction of an excessive response in in vitro fertilization from patient characteristics and ovarian reserve tests and comparison in subgroups: an individual patient data meta-analysis. Fertil Steril. 2013:100. https://doi.org/10.1016/j.fertnstert.2013.04.024.

15. Pfeifer S, Butts S, Dumesic D, Fossum G, Gracia C, La Barbera A, et al. Prevention and treatment of moderate and severe ovarian hyperstimulation syndrome: a guideline. Fertil Steril. 2016:106. https://doi.org/10.1016/j.fertnstert.2016.08.048.
16. Zegers-Hochschild F, Adamson GD, Dyer S, Racowsky C, de Mouzon J, Sokol R, et al. The international glossary on infertility and fertility care, 2017. Fertil Steril. 2017:108. https://doi.org/10.1016/j.fertnstert.2017.06.005.
17. La Marca A, Sunkara SK. Individualization of controlled ovarian stimulation in IVF using ovarian reserve markers: from theory to practice. Hum Reprod Update. 2014:20. https://doi.org/10.1093/humupd/dmt037.

The Current Status of Metformin in OHSS Prevention

9

Akanksha Kulshreshtha, Ariel Revel,
and Jennia Michaeli

9.1 Introduction

The role of metformin for ovulation induction in women with polycystic ovary syndrome (PCOS) has been well documented [1, 2]. However, its role in the prevention of ovarian hyperstimulation syndrome (OHSS) needs to be fully delineated. Over the last two decades, we have seen mixed evidence regarding the benefits of using metformin during ovarian stimulation. We will discuss the biological rationale behind the use of metformin in mitigating the risk of OHSS and current evidence in clinical practice.

A. Kulshreshtha · J. Michaeli
Department of Obstetrics and Gynaecology, University of Toronto; Mount Sinai Fertility, Toronto, ON, Canada
e-mail: akanksha.kulshreshtha@mail.utoronto.ca; Jennia.Michaeli@sinaihealth.ca

A. Revel (✉)
Director of Medical Affairs, Kadimastem, Nes-Ziona, Israel

Tel Aviv University Medical School, Tel Aviv, Israel

Hebrew University Medical School, Jerusalem, Israel

G. N. Allahbadia et al. (eds.), *Ovarian Hyperstimulation Syndrome (OHSS) Free Clinic*, https://doi.org/10.1007/978-981-95-3289-6_9

9.2 Metabolic Pathways in the Pathophysiology of OHSS

In a physiologic menstrual cycle, a small number of antral follicles are recruited by the endogenous hormonal milieu, and a single dominant follicle is selected for ovulation under the tight control of the hypothalamic-pituitary-ovarian axis feedback interaction. Conversely, during assisted reproductive technology (ART) cycles, the administration of exogenous gonadotropins drives the simultaneous recruitment of multiple antral follicles, aiming to maximize oocyte yield and pregnancy outcomes [3, 4]. Ovarian hyperstimulation syndrome (OHSS) is almost exclusively an iatrogenic complication that can be seen after ovarian stimulation in ART cycles and can potentially be lethal [3].

In women with PCOS, there is an altered pattern of gonadotropin secretion, hyperandrogenism, and insulin resistance [5]. Insulin resistance has been identified as a major factor contributing to infertility in this population [6]. The increased amount of circulating insulin levels stimulates ovarian androgen production and decreases hepatic sex hormone-binding globulin (SHBG) production, further increasing the circulating androgen levels. Generally, anti-Müllerian hormone concentrations are higher in women with PCOS, correlating with the abundance of small antral follicles. There is a potential to have an exaggerated response to stimulation due to a higher ovarian reserve and more growing follicles [5].

Although the exact pathophysiology of OHSS is not clearly understood, it is thought that the syndrome occurs as a result of multiple follicles being recruited and leading to excessive release of vasoactive peptides such as vascular endothelial growth factor (VEGF) and prostaglandins from granulosa cells in the hyperstimulated ovaries [3]. VEGF binds to the VEGFR2 receptor on endothelial cells and leads to increased vascular permeability [4, 7]. Using human chorionic gonadotropin (hCG) as an ovulatory trigger can also lead to a direct increase in VEGF production and further propagate this effect. Other pro-inflammatory cytokines such as interleukin-1β, IL-6, IL-8, and tumor necrosis factor α, as well as the mediators of the renin–angiotensin–aldosterone system, have all been implicated in the pathophysiology of OHSS. More recently, the role of AMP-activated protein kinase (AMPK) enzyme was recognized as a contributing pathway in OHSS pathogenesis [8]. The clinical outcome of these multiple pathway activations is arteriolar vasodilation and increased vascular permeability, resulting in a shift of fluid from intravascular to extravascular spaces. This shift causes hemoconcentration, hyponatremia, and hypercoagulability, which leads to impaired organ function. Symptoms can range from mild bloating due and enlarged ovaries, to renal failure and even death [3, 4].

9.3 Pharmacokinetics of Metformin

Metformin is an oral biguanide that lowers blood glucose levels by acting as an insulin sensitizer, which does not cause hypoglycemia [9]. Metformin has been used in clinical practice for over 50 years in various patient populations [10]. In the context of reproduction, it is used most commonly in women with PCOS, type 2 diabetes, and hyperglycemia [6, 9, 10]. It primarily works by reducing the absorption of glucose from the gastrointestinal tract, inhibiting the production of hepatic glucose, and increasing insulin-stimulated glucose uptake in the peripheral tissues. As a secondary action, the improved insulin levels decrease androgen production and luteinizing hormone (LH) concentrations and increase SHBG levels. It has also been suggested that metformin may act directly on theca cells in the ovaries to reduce the production of androgens [2, 11]. Additionally, in an experimental model, metformin was shown to act as an AMPK pathway inhibitor [8].

It is postulated that this reduction of ovarian hyperandrogenism reduces the number of preovulatory follicles and, thus, the risk of OHSS. In women with PCOS, metformin has been thought to improve the frequency of ovulation and menstrual cycles and improve clinical pregnancy rates [2, 6, 12].

Most studies have demonstrated that metformin administered at a dose of 500 mg three times daily regulates menstrual cycles, improves spontaneous ovulation, and promotes fertility [2].

9.4 International Consensus Regarding the Effect of Metformin on the Risk of OHSS

In 2006, a randomized trial by Tang et al. was conducted to determine the benefits of using metformin during IVF treatment. Their primary outcome was to explore improvement in fertilization rates, and their secondary outcome was to investigate the effects on pregnancy and severe OHSS. They had 101 women enrolled in the study who met the Rotterdam criteria for PCOS diagnosis—52 in the metformin group and 49 in the placebo group. This study found that metformin given during ovarian stimulation with a gonadotropin-releasing hormone (GnRH) agonist protocol increased pregnancy outcomes, such as clinical pregnancy and live birth rate, and decreased the incidence of severe OHSS in women with PCOS. However, there was no benefit of metformin treatment on fertilization rates (52.9 vs. 54.9%, $P = 0.641$) [13].

Metformin has also been shown to be beneficial not only in the obese PCOS population but also in individuals with a low BMI of <28 kg/m^2, when administered during gonadotropin stimulation. In a retrospective review by Kumbak in Turkey in 2009, it was found that metformin administrated was associated with a higher implantation and pregnancy rate [14].

Since then, additional studies have reported the decreased incidence of OHSS in women who were treated with metformin in the context of PCOS; however, the improved live birth rates have not been seen consistently [10, 11, 15]. More specifically, a double blind, placebo-controlled RCT done by Palomba et al. (2011), on 120 patients, found that in patients with PCOS who are at high risk of OHSS, metformin reduced the risk of OHSS. The total incidence of OHSS was observed to have been reduced by approximately 70% with a NNT of 5. Interestingly, there was no significant difference noted in the implantation, clinical pregnancy, and ongoing pregnancy rates between the metformin and placebo groups [11].

Current practice in the field of reproductive endocrinology has shifted to using gonadotropin-releasing hormone (GnRH) antagonist protocols, which allow for the use of a GnRH agonist trigger for final oocyte maturation [16]. In expected high responders and in women with PCOS, the introduction of the GnRH antagonist protocol has significantly decreased the incidence of moderate to severe OHSS for several reasons. Compared to the natural cycle luteinizing hormone (LH) surge that lasts approximately 48 h, the endogenous release of LH that is induced by the GnRH agonist administration is short-lived, and estimated at 28–32 h. This is radically different from the traditional human chorionic gonadotropin (hCG) trigger that has a lingering effect for up to 6–7 days. In addition to the luteolytic effect of the GnRH agonist, the improvement of oocyte cryopreservation techniques with increased success rates of oocyte vitrification and freeze-thaw cycles has promoted cycle segmentation. The introduction of GnRH agonist trigger into clinical practice, in combination with an increasing tendency for a freeze-all policy, has almost eradicated the incidence of severe OHSS and has rendered IVF a safe and effective procedure in women with PCOS [17].

Interestingly, metformin has not been thoroughly studied in combination with the GnRH antagonist protocols. One recent RCT by Jacob et al. randomized 153 patients with PCOS. In the study population, 77 patients received metformin and 76 received a placebo. The primary objective of this study was to evaluate the potential effect of metformin on the incidence of OHSS in a GnRH antagonist IVF cycle. All patients in the metformin group received a dose of 850 mg twice a day. The results found that metformin did not lead to a significant reduction in the incidence of moderate to severe OHSS compared to placebo, $p = 0.66$. Although not their primary outcome, findings of this study also suggested that metformin may reduce pregnancy rates in a GnRH antagonist cycle [18].

Based on these limited data, the various international guidelines have nonuniform clinical recommendations. The American Society of Reproductive Medicine (ASRM) and the European Society of Human Reproduction and Embryology (ESHRE) offer differing guidelines on the use of metformin for OHSS risk reduction. ASRM suggests its use in GnRH agonist protocols but not in

GnRH antagonist protocols, while ESHRE does not recommend routine use due to inconsistent evidence. This divergence underscores the need for further research to establish more uniform guidelines [19, 20].

Most recently, however, the HERA Delphi consensus statement on the management of hyper-responders undergoing IVF stated that it is unclear whether a subset of women would benefit from the addition of metformin. As a result, they recommend adding metformin before and/or during ovarian stimulation only if the patient has PCOS and is insulin resistant [21].

Based on these guidelines, it is not clear what the best practice is for metformin use in PCOS patients for OHSS risk reduction.

9.5 Recent Evidence Regarding Metformin and New Pharmacologic Agents to Prevent OHSS

A 2022 network meta-analysis by Wu et al. investigated 40 randomized controlled trials comparing nine different drug interventions for OHSS prevention, such as metformin, cabergoline, and aspirin. The analysis concluded that metformin's role and efficacy in preventing OHSS remain controversial, particularly in patients with PCOS. Specifically, metformin did not significantly reduce the incidence of moderate to severe OHSS compared to placebo ($p = 0.66$). In contrast, cabergoline showed some promise in reducing OHSS rates, highlighting the need for further research to determine the most effective prevention strategies [22].

Further, a new agent has come to light in the past few years. Inositol is a nutritional supplement that works as a second messenger through calcium signaling pathways and plays a role in insulin signaling transmission. Inositol is found in higher concentrations in reproductive organs and has nine different forms, two of which are myoinositol and D-chiro-inositol, and play an important role in mediating different actions of insulin and are known as sensitizing agents. Myoinositol is responsible for glucose uptake, and D-chiro-inositol is responsible for glycogen synthesis. Inositol is suggested to be a novel agent that may improve ovulation frequency and menstrual cycle regularity. The reason for that is that studies have revealed a decreased bioavailability of inositol in the tissues of women with PCOS, which may contribute to the insulin resistance within the population. It is generally recommended that myoinositol be given for 3 months prior to the IVF cycle [23].

There is an emerging body of evidence investigating the use of myoinositol. In a Cochrane review meta-analysis of seven studies looking at myoinositol, there was insufficient evidence about the adequacy of inositol in the PCOS population [23]. Similarly, another meta-analysis by Unanyan et al. commented on the uncertainty of the benefits of inositol use in PCOS and the need for further trials to address its usage to improve ART cycle outcomes [24]. Both meta-analyses alluded to the lack of strong-quality evidence to support the use of myoinositol in the PCOS population.

In a recent double-blinded RCT by Rajasekaran et al., myoinositol was compared to metformin in 102 women with infertility and PCOS. Myoinositol was found to be equally beneficial as metformin in reducing the risk of OHSS in women with PCOS undergoing GnRH antagonist ART cycles. Authors also commented on the benefit of fewer gastrointestinal side effects associated with inositol, which may improve long-term compliance with the treatment [25]. Further studies with larger sample sizes are required to determine the benefit of inositol in comparison to metformin and its impact on ART and live birth outcomes.

9.6 Conclusion

In ART, prevention of OHSS remains a challenge, and the role of pharmacologic agents such as metformin remains unclear. It appears that clinical interventions such as the choice to induce final follicular maturation with GnRH agonist trigger and cycle segmentation by freeze-all embryos have had a significant impact on eliminating cases of moderate to severe OHSS in the modern ART practice, minimizing the need for and use of metformin for primary OHSS prevention.

The use of metformin, and more recently, inositol, may still be beneficial in patients with PCOS to improve ovulation frequency and pregnancy outcomes. Further studies are required to fully elucidate the role of metformin and other oral agents in limiting the risk of OHSS in the diverse population of people with infertility undergoing ART.

References

1. Bordewijk EM, Nahuis M, Costello MF, Van der Veen F, Tso LO, Mol BW, et al. Metformin during ovulation induction with gonadotrophins followed by timed intercourse or intrauterine insemination for subfertility associated with polycystic ovary syndrome. Cochrane Database Syst Rev. 2017;1(1):CD009090. https://doi.org/10.1002/14651858.CD009090.pub2. PMID: 28118681; PMCID: PMC6464837.
2. Tso LO, Costello MF, Albuquerque LE, Andriolo RB, Macedo CR. Metformin treatment before and during IVF or ICSI in women with polycystic ovary syndrome. Cochrane Database Syst Rev. 2014;2014(11):CD006105. https://doi.org/10.1002/14651858.CD006105.pub3. Update in: Cochrane Database Syst Rev. 2020 Dec 21;12:CD006105. PMID: 25406011; PMCID: PMC6953331.
3. Nelson SM. Prevention and management of ovarian hyperstimulation syndrome. Thromb Res. 2017;151(Suppl 1):S61–4. https://doi.org/10.1016/S0049-3848(17)30070-1. PMID: 28262238.
4. Kwik M, Maxwell E. Pathophysiology, treatment and prevention of ovarian hyperstimulation syndrome. Curr Opin Obstet Gynecol. 2016;28(4):236–41. https://doi.org/10.1097/GCO.0000000000000284. PMID: 27273307.
5. Rushing JS, Santoro N. Fertility issues in polycystic Ovarian disease: a systematic approach. Endocrinol Metab Clin N Am. 2021;50(1):43–55. https://doi.org/10.1016/j.ecl.2020.10.004. Epub 2021 Jan 4. PMID: 33518185.
6. Kanda S, Chatha U, Odoma VA, Pitliya A, AlEdani EM, Bhangu JK, et al. Effect of metformin (MTF) intervention during pregnancy in women with polycystic Ovarian syndrome (PCOS): a systematic review. Cureus. 2023;15(8):e44166. https://doi.org/10.7759/cureus.44166. PMID: 37753037; PMCID: PMC10519644.
7. Elia EM, Quintana R, Carrere C, Bazzano MV, Rey-Valzacchi G, Paz DA, et al. Metformin decreases the incidence of ovarian hyperstimulation syndrome: an experimental study. J Ovarian Res. 2013;6(1):62. https://doi.org/10.1186/1757-2215-6-62. PMID: 24011132; PMCID: PMC3851870.

8. Kosmas IP, Kitsou C, Lazaros L, Markoula S, Peschos D, Mynbaev O, et al. Everolimus, an mTOR pathway inhibitor, is highly successful on ovarian hyperstimulation syndrome by reducing ovarian weight and progesterone levels: a preclinical experimental randomized controlled study. Gynecol Endocrinol. 2015;31(9):702–7. https://doi.org/10.3109/09513590.2015.1065479. Epub 2015 Jul 14. PMID: 26172931.
9. Wu Y, Tu M, Huang Y, Liu Y, Zhang D. Association of Metformin with Pregnancy Outcomes in women with polycystic Ovarian syndrome undergoing in vitro fertilization: a systematic review and meta-analysis. JAMA Netw Open. 2020;3(8):e2011995. https://doi.org/10.1001/jamanetworkopen.2020.11995. PMID: 32744629; PMCID: PMC7399751.
10. Du Y, Zhu YJ, Zhou YX, Ding J, Liu JY. Metformin in therapeutic applications in human diseases: its mechanism of action and clinical study. Mol Biomed. 2022;3(1):41. https://doi.org/10.1186/s43556-022-00108-w. PMID: 36484892; PMCID: PMC9733765.
11. Palomba S, Falbo A, Carrillo L, Villani MT, Orio F, Russo T, et al. Metformin reduces risk of ovarian hyperstimulation syndrome in patients with polycystic ovary syndrome during gonadotropin-stimulated in vitro fertilization cycles: a randomized, controlled trial. Fertil Steril. 2011;96(6):1384–1390.e4. https://doi.org/10.1016/j.fertnstert.2011.09.020. Epub 2011 Oct 7. PMID: 21982727.
12. Wei Z, Cao Y, Cong L, Zhou P, Zhang Z, Li J. Effect of metformin pretreatment on pregnancy outcome of in vitro matured oocytes retrieved from women with polycystic ovary syndrome. Fertil Steril. 2008;90(4):1149–54. https://doi.org/10.1016/j.fertnstert.2007.07.1385. Epub 2007 Nov 26. Retraction in: Fertil Steril. 2015 Oct;104(4):1048. PMID: 18022165.
13. Tang T, Glanville J, Orsi N, Barth JH, Balen AH. The use of metformin for women with PCOS undergoing IVF treatment. Hum Reprod. 2006;21:1416–25.
14. Kumbak B, Kahraman S. Efficacy of metformin supplementation during ovarian stimulation of lean PCOS patients undergoing in vitro fertilization. Acta Obstet Gynecol Scand. 2009;88(5):563–8.
15. Khattab S, Fotouh IA, Mohesn IA, Metwally M, Moaz M. Use of metformin for prevention of ovarian hyperstimulation syndrome: a novel approach. Reprod Biomed Online. 2006;13(2):194–7. https://doi.org/10.1016/s1472-6483(10)60614-1. PMID: 16895631.
16. Casper RF. Basic understanding of gonadotropin-releasing hormone-agonist triggering. Fertil Steril. 2015;103(4):867–9. https://doi.org/10.1016/j.fertnstert.2014.12.129. Epub 2015 Feb 21. PMID: 25712575.
17. Humaidan P, Haahr T. GnRHa trigger-the story of the ugly duckling. F S Rep. 2023;4(2 Suppl):15–9. https://doi.org/10.1016/j.xfre.2023.02.011. PMID: 37223771; PMCID: PMC10201294.

18. Jacob SL, Brewer C, Tang T, Picton HM, Barth JH, Balen AH. A short course of metformin does not reduce OHSS in a GnRH antagonist cycle for women with PCOS undergoing IVF: a randomised placebo-controlled trial. Hum Reprod. 2016;31(12):2756–64. https://doi.org/10.1093/humrep/dew268. Epub 2016 Nov 5. PMID: 27816925.
19. Practice Committee of the American Society for Reproductive Medicine. Electronic address: ASRM@asrm.org; Practice Committee of the American Society for Reproductive Medicine. Prevention and treatment of moderate and severe ovarian hyperstimulation syndrome: a guideline. Fertil Steril. 2016;106(7):1634–47. https://doi.org/10.1016/j.fertnstert.2016.08.048. Epub 2016 Sep 24. PMID: 27678032.
20. Ovarian Stimulation TEGGO, Bosch E, Broer S, Griesinger G, Grynberg M, Humaidan P, et al. ESHRE guideline: ovarian stimulation for IVF/ICSI†. Hum Reprod Open. 2020;2020(2):hoaa009. https://doi.org/10.1093/hropen/hoaa009. Erratum in: Hum Reprod Open. 2020 Dec 29;2020(4):hoaa067. PMID: 32395637; PMCID: PMC7203749.
21. Feferkorn I, Santos-Ribeiro S, Ubaldi FM, Velasco JG, Ata B, Blockeel C, et al. The HERA (Hyper-response Risk Assessment) Delphi consensus for the management of hyper-responders in in vitro fertilization. J Assist Reprod Genet. 2023;40(11):2681–95. https://doi.org/10.1007/s10815-023-02918-5. Epub 2023 Sep 15. Erratum in: J Assist Reprod Genet. 2024 Feb;41(2):519–520. PMID: 37713144; PMCID: PMC10643792.
22. Wu D, Shi H, Yu Y, Yu T, Zhai J. Comparison of the effectiveness of various medicines in the prevention of Ovarian Hyperstimulation syndrome: a network meta-analysis of randomized controlled trials. Front Endocrinol (Lausanne). 2022;26(13):808517. https://doi.org/10.3389/fendo.2022.808517. PMID: 35154015; PMCID: PMC8825486.
23. Showell MG, Mackenzie-Proctor R, Jordan V, Hodgson R, Farquhar C. Inositol for subfertile women with polycystic ovary syndrome. Cochrane Database Syst Rev. 2018;12(12):CD012378. https://doi.org/10.1002/14651858.CD012378.pub2. PMID: 30570133; PMCID: PMC6516980.
24. Unanyan A, Pivazyan L, Krylova E, Eskin A, Zakaryan A, Sarkisova A, et al. Effectiveness of inositol, metformin and their combination in women with PCOS undergoing assisted reproduction: systematic review and meta-analysis. Gynecol Endocrinol. 2022;38(12):1035–46. https://doi.org/10.1080/09513590.2022.2136160. Epub 2022 Oct 26.
25. Rajasekaran K, Malhotra N, Mahey R, Khadgawat R, Kalaivani M. Myoinositol *versus* metformin pretreatment in GnRH-antagonist cycle for women with PCOS undergoing IVF: a double-blinded randomized controlled study. Gynecol Endocrinol. 2022;38(2):140–7. https://doi.org/10.1080/09513590.2021.1981282. Epub 2021 Sep 30. PMID: 34590929.

Tweaking Follicular Phase Stimulation Protocols for Prevention of OHSS

10

Sulbha Arora and Jyoti Tripathi

10.1 Introduction

Ovarian hyperstimulation syndrome (OHSS) is one of the most serious complications associated with ovarian stimulation. Although its incidence is low, occurring in approximately 1–5% of in vitro fertilization (IVF) cycles [1–5], it can escalate into a potentially life-threatening situation. As IVF is otherwise an elective procedure, and OHSS an iatrogenic complication, strategies need to be implemented to eradicate it completely and ensure an OHSS-free clinic.

The aim of controlled ovarian stimulation (COS) during IVF is to promote the growth of multiple ovarian follicles, in order to increase the number of oocytes available during oocyte retrieval. Ovarian response to COS with gonadotropins may vary widely from patient to patient. Women have accordingly been classified as normal, low, or high responders, although there is no generally accepted consensus on the number of follicles qualifying for each category. One might think that a high ovarian response is desirable

S. Arora (✉)
Nova IVF Fertility, Mumbai, Maharashtra, India

J. Tripathi
Nova IVF Fertility, Indore, Madhya Pradesh, India

G. N. Allahbadia et al. (eds.), *Ovarian Hyperstimulation Syndrome (OHSS) Free Clinic*, https://doi.org/10.1007/978-981-95-3289-6_10

for IVF, as a higher number of oocytes would lead to a higher number of embryos, in turn leading to a better selection of good-quality embryos for transfer and thus improving reproductive outcomes. However, the live birth rates only increase proportionately with the number of retrieved oocytes up to a certain extent, beyond which they plateau. In one study, data from 7422 women who underwent their first IVF cycle showed that the highest pregnancy rates per embryo transfer and per started cycle were observed when 13 oocytes were obtained [6]. In another study, data from 77,956 fresh IVF cycles performed over a period of 6 years were extracted from The Swedish National Quality Registry of Assisted Reproduction. The results showed that live birth rates increased up to 11 oocytes retrieved and then evened out. The cumulative live birth rate per retrieval considering the fresh and all subsequent frozen transfers coming out of it increased till about 20 oocytes. A shift was seen at approximately 18 to 20 oocytes, where the cumulative delivery rates leveled off, and at the same time, the incidence of severe OHSS increased significantly [7]. During ovarian stimulation, it is therefore desirable to ensure the response remains within this cutoff in order to prevent OHSS from occurring.

An unexpected excessive response is usually the result of administering high doses of gonadotropins. However, patients' individual characteristics might account for a high ovarian response as well, regardless of the gonadotropin doses. This is especially true for patients with multifollicular ovaries or for those diagnosed with polycystic ovarian syndrome (PCOS). Women with PCOS have only a narrow boundary between the minimum effective dose of gonadotropins and doses that can suddenly induce excessive follicular growth. Even small dose modifications might induce a high ovarian response and ensuing clinical complications, of which OHSS is the most dreaded [8, 9].

Understanding the pathophysiology of this condition may aid in identifying ways to prevent its development.

10.2 Prevention of OHSS

Prevention strategies for OHSS are broadly classified as primary and secondary in nature.

Primary Prevention Primary prevention identifies women at risk of OHSS and classifies them into high, normal, or low risk. This enables the individualized selection of appropriate stimulation protocols that lead to an adequate response without hyperstimulating the ovaries.

Strategies for primary prevention include [10]:

1. Identifying patients at risk of developing OHSS.
2. Use of GnRH antagonist protocols.
3. Dosing gonadotropins based on individual patient parameters.
4. Lowering the starting dose of gonadotropins.
5. Addition of oral ovulogens to COS protocols.
6. Addition of adjuvants such as metformin in cases of PCOS.
7. Use of a GnRH agonist to trigger final oocyte maturation.

Secondary Prevention Secondary prevention focuses on methods used in patients who have already displayed an excessive response to ovarian stimulation during a cycle and aims to prevent progression to OHSS.

Strategies for secondary prevention include [10]:

1. Reducing the dose of gonadotropins depending on the number of growing follicles or serum estradiol (E_2) levels.
2. Reducing the duration of stimulation.
3. Addition of recombinant LH to a recombinant FSH-only protocols.
4. Coasting.
5. Cycle cancellation.
6. Use of a GnRH agonist trigger.
7. Elective freezing of all embryos.
8. Use of dopamine agonists such as cabergoline or GnRH antagonist injections post-trigger or post-OPU.

Primary preventive strategies have been covered in detail in other chapters of this book. This chapter focuses on the first part of secondary prevention, which is tweaking stimulation protocols during the follicular phase in order to keep the number of growing follicles, and the serum estradiol levels in check, thereby preventing the progression to OHSS.

10.3 Identifying Patients at Risk of OHSS

While any woman undergoing controlled ovarian stimulation (COS) with gonadotropins may develop ovarian hyperstimulation syndrome (OHSS), certain groups are more predisposed to this complication. The 2024 ASRM Practice Committee Guidelines on the Prevention of Moderate and Severe OHSS outline evidence-based thresholds for recognizing risk factors (see Table 10.1) [10]. Identifying patients at elevated risk is crucial for applying preventive measures aimed at reducing or avoiding the occurrence of OHSS.

Table 10.1 Risk factors for OHSS

Risk factors at baseline	Risk factors during ovarian stimulation
PCOS	>17 follicles over 10 mm at the trigger
Previous OHSS	Elevated estradiol at trigger (>3500 pg/mL)
AFC > 24	>15 oocytes retrieved
AMH level > 3.4 ng/mL	

AFC antral follicle count, *AMH* anti-Müllerian hormone, *PCOS* polycystic ovarian syndrome

From the ASRM Practice Committee Guidelines on Prevention of Moderate and Severe OHSS (2024)

10.4 Risk Factors at Baseline

Certain risk factors such as age, body mass index, or the presence of polycystic ovaries have classically been considered good predictive markers for a high response to stimulation. According to a meta-analysis published by Broer et al. [11], these clinical markers, along with the evaluation of the antral follicle count (AFC) by vaginal ultrasound, defined as the total number of follicles 2–10 mm in diameter at the beginning of stimulation, and determination of serum AMH levels, have high sensitivity and specificity to predict a high response to stimulation.

Identification of these factors before starting stimulation helps to select suitable stimulation protocols and ensure a closer monitoring of the cycle, in order to avoid OHSS.

10.5 Risk Factors during Ovarian Stimulation

During cycle monitoring, there are stimulation-related factors that need to be looked out for, which predispose to a higher risk of impending OHSS. These include a greater number of preovulatory mature follicles on the day of trigger, elevated serum estradiol levels, and obtaining a larger number of oocytes after egg retrieval.

A high number of mature follicles has consistently been predictive of OHSS risk [12–16]. Total follicle number > 17 was found to be an independent risk factor for OHSS in a retrospective case-control study performed by T Ma et al. [12] One study found the risk of OHSS to be high when there were ≥ 19 follicles measuring ≥ 11 mm [15], whereas another retrospective cohort study concluded that this cutoff was ≥ 15 follicles measuring ≥ 10 mm [16].

High serum estradiol at the time of trigger has been associated with a high risk of OHSS [17–20]. There is no consensus on the cutoff, but it varies from 3500 to 5000 pg/mL across various studies.

Recent studies have demonstrated a greater risk of OHSS when at least 15–18 oocytes were retrieved [21–23]. Steward et al. conducted an analysis of an ART registry that included 256,381 cycles, demonstrating an increased risk of OHSS without an improvement in live birth rates per cycle when >15 oocytes were retrieved [1].

10.6 Tweaking Ovarian Stimulation Protocols for Prevention of OHSS

In spite of carefully identifying at-risk women and selecting individualized stimulation protocols, an unexpected high response may still be seen during monitoring. At such times, tweaking the stimulation may be required to avoid ending up with an uncontrolled response that may lead to OHSS.

10.7 Reducing the Dose of Gonadotropins During Stimulation

Ovarian stimulation regimens should be tailored to each patient's specific profile and closely monitored to maintain both effectiveness and safety [24]. Individualized treatment involves more than just the initial choice of stimulation protocols (such as using a GnRH agonist or antagonist), the type of gonadotropin, and the starting dose. It also includes making dose modifications during the stimulation process and choosing the appropriate trigger for final oocyte maturation [25]. Therefore, personalization can occur at two key stages: when beginning a new cycle (by selecting the initial dose) and during the ongoing cycle (through dose adjustments) [26–29]. Tailoring the approach, especially in patients with a predicted or unexpected high ovarian response, may help lower the chances of OHSS and reduce the likelihood of cycle cancellation.

There is strong evidence that modifying gonadotropin doses during ovarian stimulation is a common practice in clinical settings. In fact, such adjustments were noted in up to 41% of cycles reviewed in routine ART care across the United States [30]. Patients who underwent dose changes typically had higher antral follicle counts (AFC) and anti-Müllerian hormone (AMH) levels, along with lower day 3 FSH levels, compared to those who remained on a fixed dose. Additionally, those requiring dose adjustments were more often diagnosed with PCOS.

Dose adjustments during treatment are based on monitoring of the cycle by serial ultrasounds for follicular growth, and sometimes by hormonal monitoring as well [31]. Pen injectors that enable fine-tuned dose modifications offer the added advantage of helping lower the risk of OHSS by making dose adjustments more convenient and precise [32–34].

Adjusting the FSH dose during ovarian stimulation may be particularly advantageous for specific patient populations. To fully utilize ovarian capacity, shorten the time to pregnancy, and improve cumulative live birth rates, the goal is to retrieve as many oocytes as possible without increasing the patient's risk of OHSS [22, 35]. In cases where patients unexpectedly overrespond to FSH, reducing the dose mid-cycle might help prevent OHSS [36, 37]. However, many studies focusing on dose adjustments in high responders primarily explore individualized starting doses for patients already anticipated to have a high response, making it challenging to assess the effects of dose changes in those who develop an unexpected hyper-response. For example, a retrospective cohort study looked at two ovarian stimulation approaches, both using a GnRH antagonist protocol. One group received a consistent dose of 225 IU FSH daily until trigger, while the other followed a step-down regimen: 225 IU FSH on days 1–3, 150 IU on days 4–6, and 75 IU on days 7–8, along with 200 IU of low-dose hCG continued until trigger. The group with stepwise dose reduction showed a lower rate of OHSS, although live birth data were not provided [38]. In another investigation, Aboulghar et al. found that reducing the dose before initiating coasting led to a decreased incidence of moderate OHSS and fewer cycle cancellations [39].

It remains uncertain whether modifying the gonadotropin dose during stimulation itself, or the overall cumulative dose resulting from such adjustments, has a greater impact on clinical outcomes and the risk of OHSS. Consequently, further research is needed to determine whether it is the total administered dose, the act of dose modification, or a combination of both that influences treatment safety (in terms of OHSS risk) and effectiveness (including cycle cancellation rates and reproductive success per initiated cycle).

10.8 Reducing the Duration of Stimulation

There is currently no clear agreement on the ideal timing for triggering ovulation in hyper-responders, such as women with PCOS. Research specifically addressing the criteria for determining when to administer the final oocyte maturation trigger in this group remains limited. Only a small number of studies have explored how the length of ovarian stimulation impacts outcomes in women with PCOS. In one such study, Lin et al. introduced a new concept called the "proportion of dominant follicles" (PDF) as a potential indicator to guide the timing of trigger administration in PCOS patients undergoing various stimulation protocols [40]. PDF was determined by the ratio of follicles ≥18 mm to those ≥10 mm on the day of hCG administration. Based on PDF values, cycles were categorized into three groups: group A with a PDF below 20%, group B with a moderate PDF between 20% and 40%, and group C with a PDF exceeding 40%. While good quality embryos, implantation rates, and clinical pregnancy rates (CPR) were similar across all groups, the incidence of moderate-to-severe OHSS showed a significant increase with higher PDF levels. The findings suggest that maintaining a PDF in the range of 20–40% may offer an optimal balance between minimizing OHSS risk and achieving favorable pregnancy outcomes in women with PCOS, whether using a GnRH agonist long protocol or a GnRH antagonist protocol.

10.9 RecLH Supplementation in the Late Follicular Phase

There is an argument in favor of adding recombinant LH (recLH) supplementation in the late follicular phase to protocols using recombinant FSH (recFSH) alone, in order to reduce the risk of

OHSS. Caserta et al. in 2011 conducted a study to assess the efficacy of recLH supplementation in the late follicular phase on preventing clinical OHSS and cycle cancellation due to the risk of OHSS in cycles stimulated with recFSH after triptorelin downregulation for IVF. In all, 999 patients aged ≤40 with basal FSH ≤ 12 mUI/Ml were included. They were divided into two groups: group A received 150 IU recFSH till hCG trigger, and group B received 150 IU recFSH, with the addition of 75 IU recLH from day 7 till hCG trigger. In both groups, the recFSH dose was adjusted as required from day 7 onward. Although the E_2 levels on the day of trigger were higher in group B (recFSH + recLH), the number of cycles canceled due to the risk of OHSS and the incidence of clinical OHSS were higher in group A (recFSH alone). Pregnancy rates were higher in group B [41]. However, these findings were not supported by the subsequent Cochrane Database Review by Mochtar et al. in 2017 [42]. They found no difference in the OHSS rates or the percentage of cycles canceled for prevention of the same, whether recFSH alone or in combination with recLH was used in GnRH analogue downregulated IVF cycles. More recently, Eftekhar et al. performed a literature review by searching the Med line, PubMed, Google Scholar, and Scopus databases up till June 2021. They concluded that recLH support is suggested for women at risk of OHSS as it could decrease the cancellation rate caused by the development of OHSS in these patients [43]. According to the available evidence, the addition of recLH appears to be beneficial in reducing the risk of OHSS.

10.10 Coasting

Coasting is a technique where gonadotropin administration is temporarily halted while continuing pituitary suppression using either a GnRH agonist or antagonist once estradiol levels and/or follicle count reach a potentially risky threshold. The hCG trigger is postponed until estradiol levels fall to a safer range, thereby lowering the risk of OHSS. This approach is based on the understanding that larger follicles require less FSH than smaller ones. When follicles exceed 12 mm in size, discontinuing gonadotropins allows the dominant follicles to continue maturing, while the smaller ones regress. This selective growth may help decrease the production of vasoactive substances like VEGF, contributing to reduced OHSS risk [44].

The ideal duration for coasting is still unclear. However, some limited cohort studies indicate that when coasting extends to 4 days or more, it may be associated with reduced implantation rates [45, 46]. The guidelines for implementing coasting are applicable to both GnRH agonist and antagonist protocols, and comparable IVF outcomes have been observed in both cases [47]. Earlier research has demonstrated that extending coasting beyond 3 to 4 days is linked to a notable decline in pregnancy rates [46, 48]. As a result, if estradiol levels have not begun to decline by the fourth day of coasting, it may be advisable to consider canceling the cycle.

A randomized controlled trial involving 300 women assigned participants to three groups: the first group underwent coasting for up to 3 days; the second group was given cabergoline 0.25 mg daily for 8 days following the trigger; and the third group received a combination approach—1 day of coasting along with cabergoline 0.25 mg for 8 days post-trigger. The study reported a statistically significant decrease in early moderate-to-severe OHSS when the combination strategy was used [49]. In a systematic review involving 493 patients, Delvigne and Rozenberg observed that while coasting helped lower the risk of OHSS in high-risk individuals, it did not completely eliminate the possibility [50].

Early cohort studies on coasting reported a decrease in the occurrence of OHSS, while pregnancy rates remained unaffected [51, 52]. Subsequent studies found that the reduction in OHSS with coasting was comparable to other interventions such as cryopreservation [53], albumin [54], or early unilateral follicular aspiration [55].

In their Cochrane Review of eight randomized controlled trials, D'Angelo et al. found only limited evidence suggesting that coasting was more effective than no coasting in reducing moderate-to-severe OHSS [56]. Additionally, fewer oocytes were retrieved in the coasting group, leading the authors to conclude that coasting offered no clear advantage over alternative strategies.

With the development of more effective secondary prevention methods, coasting is no longer considered the first-line approach for reducing the risk of moderate-to-severe OHSS. According to the ASRM Practice Committee, the current evidence is insufficient to support the routine use of coasting for OHSS prevention (Evidence level: C; Recommendation strength: weak). Coasting may be used in combination with cabergoline and elective embryo freezing only when other, more effective options are unavailable, as it may still offer some benefit compared to taking no action. However, the impact of coasting on pregnancy outcomes remains uncertain [10].

10.11 Conclusions

Ovarian hyperstimulation syndrome (OHSS) is a recognized complication associated with controlled ovarian stimulation. To reduce the likelihood of its occurrence, it is important to identify women who may be at higher risk prior to starting treatment and to choose stimulation protocols that are designed to lower the chances of developing OHSS. Despite the current knowledge about the etiology and pathophysiology of high ovarian response, the management of patients at high risk of OHSS still presents a challenge for physicians. Thresholds of the number of recruited follicles, the serum estradiol levels, and the number of retrieved oocytes have been identified, beyond which there is a higher risk of OHSS. Monitoring of an IVF cycle by ultrasound with or without hormone levels must keep these thresholds in mind. Adjustments may need to be made to ongoing stimulation protocols, if the response appears to be approaching these thresholds, in order to avoid crossing them. These strategies for tweaking the stimulation include reducing the dose of gonadotropins being administered, reducing the duration by giving an earlier trigger, adding recLH to a recFSH only protocol, and coasting. Their efficacy in preventing OHSS appears to be only limited as per the available evidence, however. The advent of GnRH antagonist protocols, enabling the use of the safer GnRH agonist triggers, and the excellent results with embryo vitrification, provides more successful strategies to prevent OHSS as compared to making adjustments in follicular phase stimulation alone.

References

1. Steward RG, Lan L, Shah AA, Yeh JS, Price TM, Goldfarb JM, et al. Oocyte number as a predictor for ovarian hyperstimulation syndrome and live birth: an analysis of 256,381 in vitro fertilization cycles. Fertil Steril. 2014;101:967–73.
2. Luke B, Brown MB, Morbeck DE, Hudson SB, Coddington CC 3rd, Stern JE. Factors associated with ovarian hyperstimulation syndrome (OHSS) and its effect on assisted reproductive technology (ART) treatment and outcome. Fertil Steril. 2010;94:1399–404.
3. Jayaprakasan K, Chan Y, Islam R, Haoula Z, Hopkisson J, Coomarasamy A, et al. Prediction of in vitro fertilization outcome at different antral follicle count thresholds in a prospective cohort of 1,012 women. Fertil Steril. 2012;98:657–63.
4. Kahnberg A, Enskog A, Br€annstro€m M, Lundin K, Bergh C. Prediction of ovarian hyperstimulation syndrome in women undergoing in vitro fertilization. Acta Obstet Gynecol Scand. 2009;88:1373–81.
5. Papanikolaou EG, Pozzobon C, Kolibianakis EM, Camus M, Tournaye H, Fatemi HM, et al. Incidence and prediction of ovarian hyperstimulation syndrome in women undergoing gonadotropin–releasing hormone antagonist in vitro fertilization cycles. Fertil Steril. 2006;85:112–20.
6. van der Gaast MH, Eijkemans MJC, van der Net JB, de Boer EJ, Burger CW, van Leeuwen FE, Fauser BCJM, Macklon NS. Optimum number of oocytes for a successful first IVF treatment cycle. RBM Online. 2006;13(4):476–80.
7. Magnusson Å, Källen K, Thurin-Kjellberg A, Bergh C. The number of oocytes retrieved during IVF: a balance between efficacy and safety. Hum Reprod. 2018;33(1):58–64.
8. Humaidan P, Quartarolo J, Papanikolaou EG. Preventing ovarian hyperstimulation syndrome: guidance for the clinician. Fertil Steril. 2010;94(2):389–400.
9. Tan BK, Mathur R. Management of ovarian hyperstimulation syndrome. Produced on behalf of the BFS policy and practice committee. Hum Fertil. 2013;16(3):151–9.
10. Prevention of moderate and severe hyperstimulation syndrome: a guideline. Practice Committee for the American Society of reproductive medicine. Fertil Steril. 2024;121(2):230–45.

11. Broer SL, Dolleman M, Opmeer BC, et al. AMH and AFC as predictors of excessive response in controlled ovarian hyperstimulation: a meta-analysis. Hum Reprod Update. 2011;17(1):46–54.
12. Ma T, Niu Y, Wei B, Xu L, Zou L, Che X, et al. Moderate-to-severe ovarian hyperstimulation syndrome: a-retrospective multivariate logistic regression analysis in Chinese patients. Adv Clin Exp Med. 2020;29:85–90.
13. Danninger B, Brunner M, Obruca A, Feichtinger W. Prediction of ovarian hyperstimulation syndrome by ultrasound volumetric assessment [corrected] of baseline ovarian volume prior to stimulation. Hum Reprod. 1996;11:1597–9.
14. Jayaprakasan K, Herbert M, Moody E, Stewart JA, Murdoch AP. Estimating the risks of ovarian hyperstimulation syndrome (OHSS): implications for egg donation for research. Hum Fertil (Camb). 2007;10:183–7.
15. Griesinger G, Verweij PJ, Gates D, Devroey P, Gordon K, Stegmann BJ, et al. Prediction of ovarian hyperstimulation syndrome in patients treated with corifollitropin alfa or rFSH in a GnRH antagonist protocol. PLoS One. 2016;11:e0149615.
16. Tarlatzi TB, Venetis CA, Devreker F, Englert Y, Delbaere A. What is the best predictor of severe ovarian hyperstimulation syndrome in IVF? A cohort study. J Assist Reprod Genet. 2017;34:1341–51.
17. Delvigne A, Demoulin A, Smitz J, Donnez J, Koninckx P, Dhont M, et al. The ovarian hyperstimulation syndrome in in-vitro fertilization: a Belgian multicentric study. I. Clinical and biological features. Hum Reprod. 1993;8:1353–60.
18. Lee TH, Liu CH, Huang CC, Wu YL, Shih YT, Ho HN, et al. Serum anti-Mullerian hormone and estradiol levels as predictors of ovarian hyperstimulation syndrome in assisted reproduction technology cycles. Hum Reprod. 2008;23:160–7.
19. Hendriks DJ, Klinkert ER, Bancsi LF, Looman CW, Habbema JD, te Velde ER, et al. Use of stimulated serum estradiol measurements for the prediction of hyperresponse to ovarian stimulation in in vitro fertilization (IVF). J Assist Reprod Genet. 2004;21:65–72.
20. Mai Q, Hu X, Yang G, Luo Y, Huang K, Yuan Y, et al. Effect of letrozole on moderate and severe early-onset ovarian hyperstimulation syndrome in high–risk women: a prospective randomized trial. Am J Obstet Gynecol. 2017;216(42):e1–10.
21. Chen YH, Xu XH, Wang Q, Zhang SD, Jiang LL, Zhang CL, et al. Optimum oocyte retrieved and transfer strategy in young women with normal ovarian reserve undergoing a long treatment protocol: a retrospective cohort study. J Assist Reprod Genet. 2015;32:1459–67.
22. Drakopoulos P, Blockeel C, Stoop D, Camus M, de Vos M, Tournaye H, et al. Conventional ovarian stimulation and single embryo transfer for IVF/ICSI. How many oocytes do we need to maximize cumulative live

birth rates after utilization of all fresh and frozen embryos? Hum Reprod. 2016;31:370–6.
23. Magnusson A, K€allen K, Thurin-Kjellberg A, Bergh C. The number of oocytes retrieved during IVF: a balance between efficacy and safety. Hum Reprod. 2018;33:58–64.
24. Lunenfeld B, Bilger W, Longobardi S, Alam V, D'Hooghe T, Sunkara SK. The development of gonadotropins for clinical use in the treatment of infertility. Front Endocrinol (Lausanne). 2019;10:429.
25. Fatemi H, Bilger W, Denis D, Griesinger G, La Marca A, Longobardi S, Mahony M, Yin X, D'Hooghe T. Dose adjustment of follicle-stimulating hormone (FSH) during ovarian stimulation as part of medically-assisted reproduction in clinical studies: a systematic review covering 10 years (2007-2017). Reprod Biol Endocrinol. 2021;19(1):68.
26. Lensen SF, Wilkinson J, Leijdekkers JA, La Marca A, Mol BWJ, Marjoribanks J, et al. Individualised gonadotropin dose selection using markers of ovarian reserve for women undergoing in vitro fertilisation plus intracytoplasmic sperm injection (IVF/ICSI). Cochrane Database Syst Rev. 2018;2(2):Cd012693.
27. Nelson SM. Biomarkers of ovarian response: current and future applications. Fertil Steril. 2013;99(4):963–9.
28. Sighinolfi G, Grisendi V, La Marca A. How to personalize ovarian stimulation in clinical practice. J Turk Ger Gynecol Assoc. 2017;18(3):148–53.
29. Lunenfeld B, Bilger W, Longobardi S, Kirsten J, D'Hooghe T, Sunkara SK. Decision points for individualized hormonal stimulation with recombinant gonadotropins for treatment of women with infertility. Gynecol Endocrinol. 2019;35(12):1027–36.
30. Mahony MH, B. Richter, K. D'Hooghe, T. Abstracts of the 34th annual meeting of the European Society of Human Reproduction and Embryology (P^{-659}); occurrence and characteristics of recombinant human follicle-stimulating hormone (r-hFSH) dose adjustments during ovarian stimulation in a real-world US database study of 33,962 IVF patient cycles. Hum Reprod 2018;33(suppl_1):i444.
31. Bosch E, Broer S, Griesinger G, Grynberg M, Humaidan P, Kolibianakis E, et al. ESHRE guideline: ovarian stimulation for IVF/ICSI. Hum Reprod Open. 2020;2020(2):hoaa009.
32. Olivennes F, Trew G, Borini A, Broekmans F, Arriagada P, Warne DW, Howles CM. Randomized, controlled, open-label, non-inferiority study of the CONSORT algorithm for individualized dosing of follitropin alfa. Reprod Biomed Online. 2015;30(3):248–57.
33. Yovich J, Stanger J, Hinchliffe P. Targeted gonadotrophin stimulation using the PIVET algorithm markedly reduces the risk of OHSS. Reprod Biomed Online. 2012;24(3):281–92.
34. Yovich JL, Alsbjerg B, Conceicao JL, Hinchliffe PM, Keane KN. PIVET rFSH dosing algorithms for individualized controlled ovarian stimulation

enables optimized pregnancy productivity rates and avoidance of ovarian hyperstimulation syndrome. Drug Des Devel Ther. 2016;10:2561–73.
35. Malchau SS, Henningsen AA, Forman J, Loft A, Nyboe Andersen A, Pinborg A. Cumulative live birth rate prognosis based on the number of aspirated oocytes in previous ART cycles. Hum Reprod. 2019;34(1):171–80.
36. Delvigne A, Rozenberg S. Epidemiology and prevention of ovarian hyperstimulation syndrome (OHSS): a review. Hum Reprod Update. 2002;8(6):559–77.
37. Gera PS, Tatpati LL, Allemand MC, Wentworth MA, Coddington CC. Ovarian hyperstimulation syndrome: steps to maximize success and minimize effect for assisted reproductive outcome. Fertil Steril. 2010;94(1):173–8.
38. Iaconelli CAR, Setti AS, Braga DPAF, Maldonado LGL, Iaconelli A Jr, Borges E Jr, et al. Concomitant use of FSH and low-dose recombinant hCG during the late follicular phase versus conventional controlled ovarian stimulation for intracytoplasmic sperm injection cycles. Hum Fertil (Camb). 2017;20:285–92.
39. Aboulghar MA, Mansour RT, Serour GI, Rhodes CA, Amin YM. Reduction of human menopausal gonadotropin dose before coasting prevents severe ovarian hyperstimulation syndrome with minimal cycle cancellation. J Assist Reprod Genet. 2000;17(5):298–301.
40. Lin HY, Li Y, Wang WJ, Qiu Q, Zhang QX, Li Y. Role of the proportion of dominant follicles in patients with polycystic ovary syndrome undergoing in vitro fertilization-embryo transfer. Chin Med J. 2019;132(12):1448.
41. Caserta D, Lisi F, Marci R, Ciardo F, Fazi A, Lisi R, Moscarini M. Does supplementation with recombinant luteinizing hormone prevent ovarian hyperstimulation syndrome in down regulated patients undergoing recombinant follicle stimulating hormone multiple follicular stimulation for IVF/ET and reduces cancellation rate for high risk of hyperstimulation? Gynecol Endocrinol. 2011;27(11):862–6.
42. Mochtar MH, Danhof NA, Ayeleke RO, Van der Veen F, van Wely M. Recombinant luteinizing hormone (rLH) and recombinant follicle stimulating hormone (rFSH) for ovarian stimulation in IVF/ICSI cycles. Cochrane Database Sys Rev. 2017;(5):CD005070.
43. Eftekhar M, Tabibnejad N. Recombinant luteinizing hormone supplementation in assisted reproductive technology: a review of literature. Middle East Fertil Soc J. 2021;26:37.
44. Benadiva CA, Davis O, Kigman I, Moomjy M, Liu HC, Rosenwaks Z. Withholding gonadotrophin administration is an effective alternative for the prevention of ovarian hyperstimulation syndrome. Fertil Steril. 1997;67:724–7.
45. Nardo LG, Cheema P, Gelbaya TA, Horne G, Fitzgerald CT, Pease EH, et al. The optimal length of 'coasting protocol' in women at risk of

ovarian hyperstimulation syndrome undergoing in vitro fertilization. Hum Fertil (Camb). 2006;9:175–80.
46. Mansour R, Alboulghar M, Serour G, Amin Y, Abou-Setta AM. Criteria of a successful coasting protocol for the prevention of severe ovarian hyperstimulation syndrome. Hum Reprod. 2005;20:3167–72.
47. Farhi J, Ben-Haroush A, Lande Y, Sapir O, Pinkas H, Fisch B. In vitro fertilization cycle outcome after coasting in gonadotropin-releasing hormone (GnRH) agonist versus GnRH antagonist protocols. Fertil Steril. 2009;91:377–82.
48. García-Velasco JA, Isaza V, Quea G, Pellicer A. Coasting for the prevention of ovarian hyperstimulation syndrome: much ado about nothing? Fertil Steril. 2006;85:547–54.
49. Bassiouny YA, Dakhly DMR, Bayoumi YA, Salaheldin NM, Gouda HM, Hassan AA. Randomized trial of combined cabergoline and coasting in preventing ovarian hyperstimulation syndrome during in vitro fertilization/intracytoplasmic sperm injection cycles. Int J Gynaecol Obstet. 2018;140:217–22.
50. Delvigne A, Rozenberg S. A qualitative systematic review of coasting, a procedure to avoid ovarian hyperstimulation syndrome in IVF patients. Hum Reprod Update. 2002;8(3):291–6.
51. Al-Shawaf T, Zosmer A, Hussain S, Tozer A, Panay N, Wilson C, et al. Prevention of severe ovarian hyperstimulation syndrome in IVF with or without ICSI and embryo transfer: a modified 'coasting' strategy based on ultrasound for identification of high-risk patients. Hum Reprod. 2001;16:24–30.
52. Dhont M, Van der Straeten F, De Sutter P. Prevention of severe ovarian hyperstimulation by coasting. Fertil Steril. 1998;70:847–50.
53. Gera PS, Tatpati LL, Allemand MC, Wentworth MA, Coddington CC. Ovarian hyperstimulation syndrome: steps to maximize success and minimize effect for assisted reproductive outcome. Fertil Steril. 2010;94:173–8.
54. Chen CD, Chao KH, Yang JH, Chen SU, Ho HN, Yang YS. Comparison of coasting and intravenous albumin in the prevention of ovarian hyperstimulation syndrome. Fertil Steril. 2003;80:86–90.
55. Egbase PE, Sharhan MA, Grudzinskas JG. Early unilateral follicular aspiration compared with coasting for the prevention of severe ovarian hyper-stimulation syndrome: a prospective randomized study. Hum Reprod. 1999;14:1421–5.
56. D'Angelo A, Amso NN, Hassan R. Coasting (withholding gonadotrophins) for preventing ovarian hyperstimulation syndrome. Cochrane Database Syst Rev. 2017;5:CD002811.

Luteal-Phase Strategies to Prevent Ovarian Hyperstimulation Syndrome (OHSS)

11

Sarah Zaidi

11.1 Introduction

11.1.1 Overview of Ovarian Hyperstimulation Syndrome (OHSS)

Despite being reported in more than 60 years age, ovarian hyperstimulation syndrome (OHSS) continues to be a serious complication. This is a rare but potentially serious condition associated with ovarian stimulation through the use of gonadotropins, particularly in cycles of in vitro fertilization (IVF) [1]. Although OHSS is recognized as a disorder of the early luteal phase, it is generally initiated during the later stages of ovarian stimulation and is exacerbated by pregnancy. In light of this, prevention of OHSS during the luteal phase has become an important aspect in reducing its overall incidence and severity [2].

S. Zaidi (✉)
Indira IVF, Dadar, Mumbai, India

G. N. Allahbadia et al. (eds.), *Ovarian Hyperstimulation Syndrome (OHSS) Free Clinic*, https://doi.org/10.1007/978-981-95-3289-6_11

11.1.2 Importance of Preventing OHSS During the Luteal Phase

OHSS is a potentially serious iatrogenic complication of controlled ovarian stimulation. It is the third leading cause of hospitalization following IVF treatment. The syndrome is associated with increased capillary permeability and a fluid shift from the intravascular space to the third space. Measures to prevent OHSS should be aimed at reducing the risk throughout the stimulation phase but should also consider the increased risk in women who have become pregnant following treatment. With nearly a fifth of women attending IVF treatment developing some form of OHSS and the potentially serious morbidity of the syndrome, prevention should be of paramount concern to the clinician [3].

11.2 Pathophysiology of OHSS

OHSS has been the subject of extensive research; however, the pathophysiology of the condition is still up for debate. Previously, it was reported that estradiol (E2) concentration in serum has a significant role in the development of OHSS. Increased levels of E2 were reported in a majority of OHSS patients. Instances of OHSS, on the other hand, have been documented in patients who have low E2 levels. The most recent research indicates that VEGF has a key role in the development of OHSS. The ascitic fluid collected from women with OHSS demonstrated an elevation in vascular permeability, suggesting the involvement of vascular endothelial growth factor (VEGF) in the pathogenesis of OHSS. On the other hand, incubation with rhVEGF antiserum resulted in a considerable decrease in the intensity of the VP activity [4].

Increased secretion of hCG from the ovulation trigger induces a systemic effect on the body's capillary wall function by increasing vascular endothelial growth factor (VEGF). This increase in permeability is more pronounced in women who are pregnant as there is already a physiological increase in VEGF at the time of conception. This is why OHSS tends to be more severe and occurs earlier in pregnancy. VEGF is also secreted by theca interstitial cells and is upregulated by hCG. The interaction between hCG and VEGF at both the capillary wall level and at the intracellular autocrine/paracrine level is thought to be the key factor in the development of OHSS [5].

11.3 Risk Factors for OHSS

11.3.1 Hormonal Stimulation Protocols

Hormonal stimulation to induce follicular growth and oocyte maturation is the first step in many IVF treatment cycles, and it is this part of the treatment which greatly increases the risk of OHSS. Strategies using gonadotrophin-releasing hormone agonist (GnRH-a) as a substitute for hCG to trigger ovulation are generally seen as the most effective method for preventing OHSS. Any possibility of delayed patient start or cycle cancellation should patients not respond as expected with these methods is also considered to be an unnecessary risk factor for OHSS development [6].

11.3.2 Polycystic Ovary Syndrome (PCOS)

Shared etiologies of PCOS and OHSS lead to its increased incidence under varied presentations. PCOS is a common disorder that affects women of reproductive age and is characterized by chronic anovulation and hyperandrogenism with additional features including polycystic ovaries and insulin resistance. In addition, in women with PCOS, an increased ratio of LH:FSH produced by pituitary resistance to feedback suppression by gonadal steroids is reported. This change in the LH:FSH ratio is also a documented etiological factor of OHSS. The prolonged half-life of hCG provides an increased stimulus for ovarian follicular and luteal androgen biosynthesis. The VEGF production also increased, resulting in increased vascular permeability and ascites portraying the similar pathogenesis of OHSS induced by hCG trigger and PCOS [7].

11.3.3 Young Age and Low Body Mass Index (BMI)

The midcycle rise in the luteinizing hormone (LH) initiates the process of ovulation. It is through the binding of LH to a particular LH receptor in the granulosa cells that the hormone exerts its impact. This binding causes an increase in the production of steroids and also encourages the maturation of the cells. LH also induces the production of VEGF, cytokines, and prostaglandins in the granulosa cells. This process is regulated by the expression of the LH receptor on the granulosa cells. Hyperstimulation protocols cause an increase in the granulosa cell LH receptor, thus increasing the response to LH. This in turn augments estrogen production, which induces the upregulation of VEGF mRNA in the luteal cells. High estrogen levels are seen during early pregnancy, and it is these higher levels that are a risk factor for severe OHSS [8].

Young women have a higher risk of developing OHSS. This is partly due to a higher response to exogenous administration of gonadotrophins, leading to an increased incidence of multiple ovulation, and therefore a higher risk of developing OHSS. OHSS is seen in all age groups, but its severity is increased in younger women. Also, women with lower BMI require less exogenous FSH to stimulate the development of multiple follicles, and many studies have shown that low BMI is an independent risk factor for OHSS, due to the reduction in heparin binding protein concentration in the granulosa cells and thus a higher response to hCG [9].

11.4 Understanding the Luteal Phase

11.4.1 Definition and Duration of the Luteal Phase

The thickening of the uterine walls in preparation for pregnancy takes place during the luteal phase of the menstrual cycle, which follows the release of the egg from the ovaries. This is followed by a decline in uterine preparation if fertilization does not occur. The luteal phase ends if implantation of a fertilized egg does not occur. Due to no hCG being present, the corpus luteum degenerates and the levels of hormones decrease, discontinuing its action on the current cycle. This signifies the end of the luteal phase, as well as the end of the menstrual cycle. Its duration is around 14 days from ovulation till the beginning of the next menstrual period [10].

11.4.2 Role of Progesterone in the Luteal Phase

The actions of progesterone are at their peak during the luteal phase and are mainly on uterine preparation for embryo implantation. Should fertilization occur, production of hCG by the embryo will maintain the corpus luteum, causing it to persist and continue hormonal production. If the hormone levels drop, its action on the luteal phase will end. The pregnancy will then be upheld by progesterone levels from the placenta. Estrogen and progesterone during the luteal phase also inhibit the production of new eggs. This creates a negative feedback cycle on FSH and LH, preventing maturation of another possible egg and therefore preventing multiple pregnancies [11].

11.5 Strategies for Preventing OHSS in the Luteal Phase

11.5.1 Individualized Hormonal Stimulation Protocols

The luteal phase of the natural menstrual cycle is the standard paradigm for the clinical application of assisted reproductive technologies (ART). However, in stimulated cycles, the process of triggering oocyte maturation and the hormonal environment that follows is quite different from the natural cycle. Strategies aimed at replacing hCG for triggering final oocyte maturation and developing the appropriate luteal-phase hormonal environment could all but eliminate the incidence of OHSS in stimulated cycles [12].

The "flare effect" is caused by peripheral administration of a GnRH agonist and results in the release of FSH and LH from pituitary gonadotrophs. The term "short protocol" refers to the use of GnRH antagonist medication in IVF. It has been demonstrated that implementing this routine over the "long" treatment lowers the risk of OHSS [13].

11.5.2 GnRH Agonist

The gonadotrophin-releasing hormone agonist (GnRH-a) triggers a significant reduction in or all but eliminates the risk of OHSS in high-risk women (those with ≥20 follicles or E2 levels >3000 pg/mL). This is due to the ability of GnRH-a to completely down-regulate the pituitary, thereby preventing the endogenous LH surge. The LH surge is a key precipitant in the increased vascular permeability seen in OHSS and mediates its effects via the upregulation of VEGF [14].

11.5.3 Freeze-All Embryo Strategy

Embryo cryopreservation (EC) is the most effective method of preventing the onset of severe OHSS. EC allows for the complete withdrawal of the hormonal effects, thus enabling a total 'freeze' of the cycle. As such, it has allowed high-risk patients the option of safe continuation of the pregnancy in a future cycle [2].

11.5.4 Progesterone Supplementation in the Luteal Phase

Successful implantation depends on the embryo and endometrial receptivity coordinating as best they can, and research indicates that progesterone can effectively trigger this process. Progesterone supplementation for lipopolysaccharide (LPS) can be accessed in natural formulation (micronized) or in synthetic forms (17 alpha-hydroxy derivatives), and it can be administered subcutaneously (SC), sublingually (IM), intravaginally (IV), orally, or transdermally [15].

High-dose estradiol and progesterone in luteal support have been proposed as a means of preventing the abnormal corpora luteal function observed following the administration of a GnRH agonist trigger. Exogenous progesterone supplementation has often been shown to boost the luteal phase; however, the best way to provide progesterone is still up for debate [15].

11.5.5 Dopamine Agonists

Cabergoline is a dopamine agonist that has been shown to successfully lower the incidence of mild to moderate OHSS, without having any discernible impact on the rates of clinical pregnancy and miscarriage. It was also reported that cabergoline is effective in reducing the rate of mild OHSS; however, in severe OHSS, there is no significant effect. Therefore, it is advised to provide oral cabergoline at a dose of 0.5 mg for 8 days, beginning on the day of hCG triggering [16].

11.5.6 Albumin

Administering albumin intravenously is recommended for the prevention of OHSS. Albumin is believed to hinder the production of other substances that can potentially lead to OHSS and prevent the release of vasoactive molecules from the corpus luteum. In addition, albumin's oncotic action plays a role in preserving the volume of blood vessels and preventing the development of pleural effusion, hypovolemia, hemoconcentration, and ascites [17].

11.5.7 Other Medications

Recently, letrozole has been suggested as a useful strategy for the syndrome's prevention. As a nonsteroidal aromatase inhibitor, letrozole blocks human aromatase in a strong, selective, and reversible manner, preventing the conversion of androgens into estrogens. Letrozole administration during the luteal phase may also lessen the syndrome-related thrombosis risk. The corpus luteum pathway appears to be a reasonable theory, as patients on letrozole have shorter luteal phases and lower serum VEGF levels. Thus, a new avenue in the treatment of this illness may be opened by using letrozole following oocyte retrieval to assist lower estrogen and VEGF concentrations and maybe reduce the prevalence of OHSS. The study that is being given in this context suggests using letrozole as a medical preventive strategy for OHSS [18].

11.5.8 Vasopressin-Induced Blockage of VEGF Secretion

Relcovaptan is a non-peptide antagonist of the vasopressin receptor that can be used to modify the proliferation and vasoconstriction of vascular smooth muscle in order to limit VEGF. In a rat model, this drug has been shown to be effective in reducing the accumulation of peritoneal fluid and decreased weight gain [16].

11.6 Monitoring and Adjusting Treatment

11.6.1 Ultrasound Monitoring of Follicular Development

Regular monitoring of ovarian response is a critical component of an OHSS prevention strategy. Ideally, the risk for the development of OHSS becomes evident during the follicular phase based on the number of developing follicles and estradiol levels. Ultrasound monitoring of follicular development has become a standard practice when treating patients with ovulation induction therapy. This technique is employed in several assisted reproductive technology (ART) procedures, including in vitro fertilization and embryo transfer. The primary objective is to mitigate the likelihood of high-order multiple gestations and OHSS [19].

11.6.2 Serum Hormone Level Monitoring

Other hormonal biomarkers that have been found by research may potentially be used to assess the risk of OHSS. It has been demonstrated that baseline anti-Müllerian hormone (AMH) levels predict OHSS. In the past, oversensitivity to hCG, shown by high or quickly rising blood E2 levels on the day of the hCG trigger, was thought to be a predictor of OHSS. Serum E2 levels and follicle count together have a high sensitivity and specificity in predicting OHSS. Even though E2 levels aren't a reliable indicator of OHSS on their own, secondary OHSS prevention techniques are frequently based on them and regularly monitored [20].

11.7 Conclusion

OHSS is currently the most serious iatrogenic condition that is associated with ovulation induction and is the most important life-threatening complication of assisted reproduction. The clinical spectrum of OHSS can vary from mild to moderate forms that are a nuisance and cause discomfort, to more severe forms that can be complicated by marked ascites, hydrothorax, electrolyte imbalances, renal failure, thromboembolic phenomena, and even death. Although the mild form usually resolves spontaneously with the onset of menses, more severe cases can last several weeks and may necessitate hospital admission. It is thus essential that strategies to prevent OHSS be developed and, if possible, be individualized to suit the patient's needs and risk factors.

References

1. Schirmer DA, Kulkarni AD, Zhang Y, Kawwass JF, Boulet SL, Kissin DM. Ovarian hyperstimulation syndrome after assisted reproductive technologies: trends, predictors, and pregnancy outcomes. Fertil Steril. 2020;114(3):567–78.
2. Pakhomov SP, Orlova VS, Verzilina IN, Sukhih NV, Nagorniy AV, Matrosova AV. Risk factors and methods for predicting ovarian

Hyperstimulation syndrome (OHSS) in the in vitro fertilization. Arch Razi Inst. 2021;76(5):1461–8.
3. Rotshenker-Olshinka K, Badeghiesh A, Volodarsky-Perel A, Steiner N, Suarthana E, Dahan MH. Trends in ovarian hyperstimulation syndrome hospitalization rates in the USA: an ongoing concern. Reprod Biomed Online. 2020;41(3):357–60.
4. Grossman LC, Michalakis KG, Browne H, Payson MD, Segars JH. The pathophysiology of ovarian hyperstimulation syndrome: an unrecognized compartment syndrome. Fertil Steril. 2010;94(4):1392–8.
5. Smitz J, Platteau P. Influence of human chorionic gonadotrophin during ovarian stimulation: an overview. Reprod Biol Endocrinol. 2020;18(1):80.
6. Bourdon M, Peigné M, Solignac C, Darné B, Languille S, Pocate-Cheriet K, et al. Gonadotropin-releasing hormone agonist (alone or combined with human chorionic gonadotropin) vs. human chorionic gonadotropin alone for ovulation triggering during controlled ovarian stimulation for in vitro fertilization/intracytoplasmic sperm injection: a systematic review and meta-analysis. FS Rev. 2021;2(4):353–70.
7. Daghestani MH, Daghestani MH, Warsy A, El-Ansary A, Omair MA, Omair MA, et al. Adverse effects of selected markers on the metabolic and endocrine profiles of obese women with and without PCOS. Front Endocrinol [Internet]. 2021 [cited 2024 Apr 25];12. Available from: https://www.frontiersin.org/journals/endocrinology/articles/10.3389/fendo.2021.665446/full.
8. Papapanou M, Syristatidi K, Gazouli M, Eleftheriades M, Vlahos N, Siristatidis C. The effect of stimulation protocols (GnRH Agonist vs. Antagonist) on the activity of mTOR and Hippo pathways of ovarian Granulosa cells and its potential correlation with the outcomes of in vitro fertilization: a hypothesis. J Clin Med. 2022;11(20):6131.
9. Sun B, Ma Y, Li L, Hu L, Wang F, Zhang Y, et al. Factors Associated with Ovarian Hyperstimulation Syndrome (OHSS) Severity in Women With Polycystic Ovary Syndrome Undergoing IVF/ICSI. Front Endocrinol [Internet]. 2020 [cited 2024 Apr 25];11. Available from: https://www.ncbi.nlm.nih.gov/pmc/articles/PMC7851086/.
10. Tesarik J, Conde-López C, Galán-Lázaro M. Mendoza-Tesarik R. Luteal Phase in Assisted Reproductive Technology. Front Reprod Health [Internet]. 2020 Dec 7 [cited 2024 Apr 25];2. Available from: https://www.frontiersin.org/articles/10.3389/frph.2020.595183.
11. Duncan WC. The inadequate corpus luteum. Reprod Fertil. 2021;2(1):C1–7.
12. Sciorio R, Cariati F, Fleming S, Alviggi C. Exploring the impact of controlled ovarian stimulation and non-invasive oocyte assessment in ART treatments. Life. 2023;13(10):1989.
13. El Tokhy O, Kopeika J, El-Toukhy T. An update on the prevention of ovarian hyperstimulation syndrome. Womens Health. 2016;12(5):496–503.

14. Castillo JC, Haahr T, Martínez-Moya M, Humaidan P. Gonadotropin-releasing hormone agonist for ovulation trigger—OHSS prevention and use of modified luteal phase support for fresh embryo transfer. Ups J Med Sci. 2020;125(2):131–7.
15. Dashti S, Eftekhar M. Luteal-phase support in assisted reproductive technology: an ongoing challenge. Int J Reprod Biomed. 2021;19(9):761–72.
16. Namavar Jahromi B, Parsanezhad ME, Shomali Z, Bakhshai P, Alborzi M, Moin Vaziri N, et al. Ovarian Hyperstimulation syndrome: a narrative review of its pathophysiology, risk factors, prevention, classification, and management. Iran J Med Sci. 2018;43(3):248–60.
17. Smith V, Osianlis T, Vollenhoven B. Prevention of ovarian Hyperstimulation syndrome: a review. Obstet Gynecol Int. 2015;2015:514159.
18. Di Guardo F, Lello C, Incognito GG, Bruno MT, Palumbo M. Letrozole and ovarian Hyperstimulation syndrome (OHSS): a promising prevention strategy. J Clin Med. 2023;12(2):614.
19. Smith LP. Ultrasound and ovarian Hyperstimulation syndrome. In: Stadtmauer LA, Tur-Kaspa I, editors. Ultrasound imaging in reproductive medicine: advances in infertility work-up, treatment and ART [internet]. Cham: springer international publishing; 2019 [cited 2024 Apr 25]. pp. 321–33. Available from: https://doi.org/10.1007/978-3-030-16699-1_19.
20. Fiedler K, Ezcurra D. Predicting and preventing ovarian hyperstimulation syndrome (OHSS): the need for individualized not standardized treatment. Reprod Biol Endocrinol RBE. 2012;10:32.

Interventional Rescue Strategies for Unexpected OHSS

12

Madhuri Patil

Key Points
- Early diagnosis and identification of comorbidities and complications to provide effective care.
- Prevent progression to severe OHSS.
- Stringent ultrasound and laboratory monitoring when OHSS is identified.
- Reduce the dose of gonadotrophin and administer GnRH agonist trigger if a GnRH antagonist protocol is used or use low-dose hCG or Rec LH if a GnRH agonist protocol is used for downregulation.
- Start the dopamine agonist on the day of the hCG trigger.
- Post-retrieval plan: freeze-all strategy.
- Administer volume expanders—albumin or hydroxyethyl starch, the latter being safer as not a blood-derived product.
- Supportive treatment—maintaining hydration, strict surveillance and monitoring, thromboprophylaxis, and paracentesis.
- Hospitalization is required for severe and critical OHSS.

M. Patil (✉)
Dr Patil's Fertility and Endoscopy Clinic, Bangalore, India

G. N. Allahbadia et al. (eds.), *Ovarian Hyperstimulation Syndrome (OHSS) Free Clinic*, https://doi.org/10.1007/978-981-95-3289-6_12

12.1 Introduction

Ovarian hyperstimulation syndrome (OHSS) is a serious, detrimental, and unintended consequence of controlled ovarian stimulation (COS) due to excessive ovarian stimulation or ovarian response to COS or hCG used for triggering ovulation [1]. The incidence of moderate and severe forms of OHSS may occur in 3–10% of all ART cycles, and may be as high as 20% among high-risk women [2].

The trigger with human chorionic gonadotropin (hCG) in patients with an excessive response [3] may increase the expression of the cystic fibrosis transmembrane conductance regulator, leading to a massive shift of body fluids through epithelial ion channels into the extravascular compartments, leading to intravascular dehydration and ascites. This is the result of sustained luteotropic activity, as hCG has a longer half-life compared to endogenous luteinizing hormone (LH) surge, which in turn causes vasodilation, increased capillary permeability, and fluid shift from intravascular to extravascular spaces, which can then result in hypovolemic hyponatremia [4]. There is also evidence of increased secretion of inflammatory mediators, like vascular endothelial growth factor (VEGF) and activation of the renin-angiotensin system in women with OHSS, which are key molecules that result in arteriolar vasodilation and increased vascular permeability [5]. The production of VEGF significantly increases after administration of hCG. Upregulation of amphiregulin (AREG) by hCG, in turn, upregulates the secretion of VEGF [6]. These pathophysiological processes can result in certain clinal sequelae like thromboembolism (1–10%), renal dysfunction (30%), adult respiratory distress syndrome (ARDS) (10–12%), or liver dysfunction (25%).

There are two primary classifications of OHSS, the first is based on the timing of presentation, and the second is based on the severity of symptoms and signs. Early OHSS generally occurs 3–7 days after hCG administration and appears to be associated with an excessive ovarian response to gonadotropin stimulation. On the contrary, the late OHSS typically occurs 12–17 days after hCG injection is more severe and requires more hospitalization, mostly always occurs in relation to pregnancy and may be associated with multiple pregnancies [7].

We can classify OHSS into four categories according to the severity of symptoms and signs [1] as shown in Table 12.1.

OHSS can be prevented by identifying high-risk patients and cycles, using low-risk treatment, and taking specific measures in individual cases. Early OHSS can be easily prevented, but not late-onset OHSS, which is related to the endogenous rise in hCG due to pregnancy. Therefore, identifying risk factors is very important when stimulating a patient with gonadotropins.

Table 12.1 OHSS—classification of severity

Mild	Moderate	Severe	Critical
Abdominal bloating/ discomfort	Moderate abdominal pain	Clinical ascites	Low blood/central venous pressure
Mild pain	Ultrasound evidence of ascites	Severe abdominal pain	Severe abdominal pain
Mild nausea/vomiting/ diarrhea	Nausea/vomiting/ diarrhea	Intractable nausea/vomiting	Rapid weight gain (>1 kg in 24 hours)
Enlarged ovaries but <8 cm	Ovaries usually 8–12 cm	Ovaries usually >12 cm	Ovaries usually >12 cm
–	Hemoconcentration (Hct >41%) Elevated WBC (>15,000 mL)	Hemoconcentration (Hct >45%, WBC >25,000/ml) Creatinine clearance <50 mL/min; Creatinine >1.6 mg/dL $Na^+ < 135$ mEq/L; $K^+ > 5$ mEq/L	Worsening of laboratory parameters
–		Hydrothorax Severe dyspnea Oliguria, liver dysfunction (elevated liver enzymes)	Syncope Pleural effusion Anuria/acute renal failure Arrhythmia Pericardial effusion and massive hydrothorax Arterial thrombosis Venous thrombosis with thromboembolism Adult respiratory distress syndrome Sepsis

12.2 Interventions for Unexpected Ovarian Hyperstimulation Syndrome (OHSS) (Fig. 12.1)

The treatment options are based on the potential risk for OHSS in women. In those at high risk of OHSS, a gonadotropin-releasing hormone (GnRH) agonist trigger followed by elective frozen embryo transfer is usually recommended [8]. For women at intermediate risk of OHSS, or those who develop unexpected OHSS, an individualized treatment approach should be considered based on the clinical and biochemical parameters.

Diagnosing unexpected OHSS is based on the number of follicles on the day of the trigger or the oocytes retrieved. According

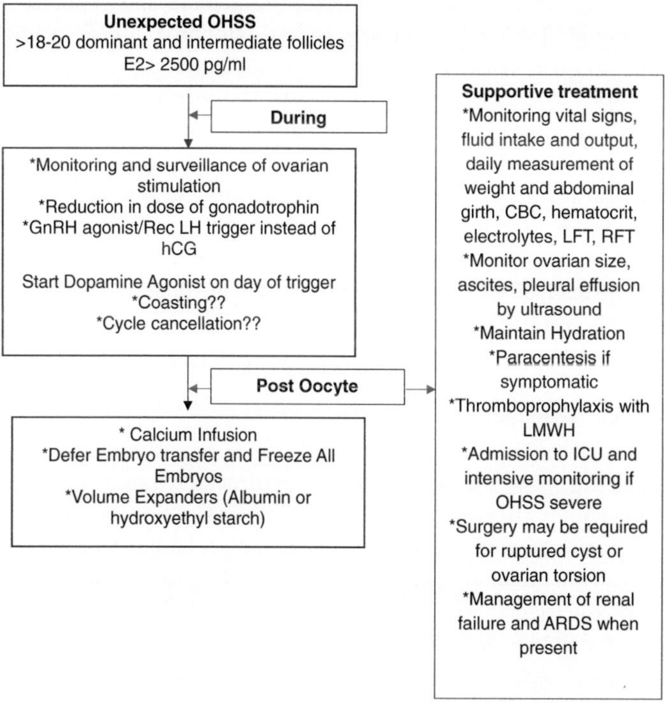

Fig. 12.1 Algorithm for the management of unexpected OHSS

to the European Society of Human Reproduction and Embryology (ESHRE), American Society for Reproductive Medicine (ASRM), and International Committee for Monitoring Assisted Reproductive Technology (ICMART), the presence of more than18–20 large or medium sized follicles and emergence of large number of small and intermediate sized follicles (10–14 mm) follicles on the day of ovulation triggering, or retrieval of more than 18–20 oocytes, may be considered as high risk for the development of OHSS in the absence of identifiable risk factors [8, 9]. The risk factors include a young lean patient with a BMI < 18 kg/m^2, AMH of >5 ng/mL, AFC of >24, and a history of previous high response to ovarian stimulation and active mutation of the FSH receptor, or LH/hCG receptors [9–11].

Interventions for unexpected ovarian hyperstimulation syndrome (OHSS) can be classified as immediate and supportive treatment. Immediate actions include stopping gonadotropin injections, increasing fluid intake with electrolyte-rich drinks, closely monitoring vital signs, performing abdominal ultrasound monitoring, considering paracentesis to drain excess abdominal fluid in severe cases, and in some situations, using medications like cabergoline to reduce fluid accumulation; for prevention in future cycles, strategies like embryo freezing, adjusting gonadotropin dosage, and using a GnRH agonist trigger instead of hCG may be implemented, depending on the severity of OHSS.

12.3 Immediate Actions

Coasting (low- or very low-quality evidence): Coasting could be considered, whereby gonadotrophin administration is withheld and hCG ovulation triggering is delayed especially in GnRH agonist downregulation cycles where a GnRH agonist cannot be given for trigger [12]. Today, with the use of GnRH antagonist protocol in most patients, this procedure has become obsolete.

Cycle Cancellation (low- or very low-quality evidence): Immediately stop any further gonadotrophin stimulation or withhold hCG once OHSS is suspected [13]. Today, with the use of individualized stimulation regimens, usually cycle cancellation is not the line of treatment adopted.

Monitoring and Surveillance of Ovarian Stimulation (low-quality evidence) [14]: Multifollicular development and elevated oestradiol levels are established predictors of OHSS development [9]. Patients with an unexpected high ovarian response to ovarian stimulation should be closely monitored with ultrasound assessment of follicular development and oestradiol (E2) levels to help in deciding the further course of treatment [15].

Reduction in Gonadotrophin Dose (low to very low-quality evidence): Excessive follicular development or a high oestradiol level may require dose reduction to prevent OHSS. This method was more commonly used in women who are young with a high ovarian reserve and those who undergo stimulation with GnRH agonist downregulation. [15–17] The gonadotrophin dose can be adjusted based on ovarian response on days 5–6 of stimulation by monitoring folliculogenesis and oestradiol levels.

GnRH Agonist Ovulation Trigger (moderate-quality evidence): GnRH agonist ovulation triggering in a GnRH antagonist cycle is recommended for women at high risk of OHSS with a freeze-all strategy, and transfer of embryos in the subsequent cycle is associated with a significantly lower risk of moderate-to-severe OHSS compared with an hCG trigger in women who unexpectedly develop more dominant and intermediate-sized follicles [8, 18]. But GnRH agonist trigger is associated with lower live birth and ongoing pregnancy rates, and an increase in early miscarriage rates if a fresh transfer is done [18].

Use of r-LH for Trigger (very low-quality evidence): A single dose of up to 30,000 IU is effective for inducing final follicular maturation with a significant reduction in OHSS [19]. When compared to hCG, there were no differences in the live birth and ongoing pregnancy rates, clinical pregnancy rate, miscarriage rate, and the number of oocytes retrieved [20].

Freeze-all Strategy (moderate-quality evidence): Embryo freezing strategy in patients with unexpectedly high ovarian response will help to substantially reduce the risk of late-onset OHSS and improve clinical outcomes when GnRH agonist trigger is administered in a GnRH antagonist protocol cycle [8].

Dopamine Agonists (moderate-quality evidence): Administration of dopamine agonists like oral cabergoline 0.5 mg daily for 8 days or bromocriptine 2.5 mg daily for 14 days or quinagolide 150 mg daily for 15 days beginning on the day of hCG administration probably reduces the incidence of moderate-to-severe OHSS compared with placebo or no intervention in women at high risk of developing OHSS [21]. The decrease in the incidence of OHSS is due to reduced neovascularization and vascular permeability as the dopamine agonist binds to dopaminergic receptors, promoting endocytosis of the VEGF receptor [21]. No difference was observed in the live birth, clinical pregnancy, and miscarriage rates. [21] There is no data to date on adverse events and pregnancy outcomes like clinical pregnancy rate, live birth rate, and miscarriage rate following treatment with a dopamine agonist.

Calcium Infusion (low or very low-quality evidence): Intravenous calcium gluconate 10%, 10 mL in 200 mL of physiologic saline, administered every day for 4 days beginning on the day of ovum pickup, may prevent OHSS. However, its regular use in the prevention of OHSS requires further research and high-quality trials [22, 23]. Calcium gluconate infusion increases serum calcium levels, which may inhibit cyclic adenosine monophosphate (cAMP)-stimulated renin secretion, decrease the production of angiotensin-converting enzyme II synthesis, and reduce VEGF expression in human luteinized granulosa cells [24]. There was no difference seen in its effectiveness as compared to dopamine agonists in preventing OHSS. There was also no difference in live birth, clinical pregnancy, and miscarriage rates between the two groups [21, 24].

Diosmin (very low-quality evidence): This natural flavonoid has anti-inflammatory and antioxidant actions and can be effectively used for reducing both the incidence of moderate-to-severe OHSS and the severity of OHSS [25]. When compared to cabergoline, its use showed no difference in the risk of occurrence of OHSS. There were also no differences seen in the clinical pregnancy and miscarriage rates [21].

Volume Expanders Albumin and hydroxyethyl starch (HES) infusion (low- or very low-quality evidence): Current evidence on the efficacy of albumin to prevent OHSS is still inconclusive. Albumin has a low molecular weight and an average half-life of 20 days. Its binding and transportation have been hypothesized to play a role in OHSS prevention by increasing the plasma oncotic pressure, which reduces the permeability effects of angiotensin II. It may also bind to vasoactive substances, related to the renin-angiotensin system and VEGF, thereby reducing platelet aggregation and blood coagulation. One meta-analysis demonstrated lower pregnancy rates after the use of albumin but not with hydroxyethyl starch infusion [26]. Today, the use of albumin is limited as it is a blood-derived product and may lead to allergic reactions, anaphylaxis, and the transmission of viral or unidentified diseases [26].

Glucocorticoid Administration (very low-quality evidence): Current research suggests that glucocorticoids are not effective in preventing OHSS and their routine use in patients with unexpected OHSS is not recommended [27].

12.4 Supportive Treatment

If OHSS prevention strategies prove ineffective, with ensuing severe OHSS, fluid resuscitation, stringent monitoring, supportive care, paracentesis, and prophylactic anticoagulation are recommended.

Hydration Encourage increased fluid intake, particularly electrolyte-rich beverages, to prevent dehydration. Fluid intake should be guided by thirst, and this is the most physiological approach to reduce intravascular dehydration. In patients showing haemoconcentration despite fluid replacement, one should use volume expanders and intravenous fluids. Diuretics should be avoided unless there is severe oliguria despite proper fluid replacement and paracentesis [28].

Monitoring Closely monitor vital signs, abdominal girth, and urine output through regular check-ups post-oocyte retrieval is necessary. A multidisciplinary approach may be necessary in the presence of critical OHSS with severe haemoconcentration and dehydration with invasive monitoring. An intensive care unit admission may be necessary [14]. Perform frequent abdominal ultrasounds to assess the extent of ovarian enlargement and free fluid in the abdomen. In the presence of severe ascites and dyspnoea, one should also rule out pleural effusion.

Hospitalization Hospitalization may be necessary in the presence of pain without satisfactory pain control with analgesics, unable to maintain adequate fluid intake due to nausea, symptoms and signs worsen despite outpatient management, the presence of respiratory distress or when a patient has critical OHSS. In severe cases with complications like respiratory distress, hospitalization with intravenous fluids and close monitoring may be required [29]. A multidisciplinary approach is best for the care of women with critical OHSS and severe OHSS who have persistent haemoconcentration and dehydration. Critical OHSS management and treatment require admission to the intensive care unit. Women with persistent haemoconcentration despite volume replacement with intravenous colloids and hydration need invasive monitoring with venous pressure and wedge pressure measurements. The patient may need extra oxygenation and should be managed with anaesthetic input. Diuretics should be avoided as they further deplete intravascular volume, but they may have a role in a multidisciplinary setting if oliguria persists despite adequate fluid replacement and drainage of ascites.

Thromboprophylaxis Thromboembolism is a potentially life-threatening complication of OHSS and, therefore, thromboprophylaxis with low-molecular-weight heparin (LMWH) at a dose of 40 mg should be considered for patients who develop severe OHSS [30, 31].

Paracentesis Paracentesis is the single most important treatment modality in life-threatening OHSS not controlled by medical therapy. It can be done both on an outpatient basis or after hospitalization. It can be done either transabdominally or transvaginally under ultrasound guidance [32]. The amount of fluid drainage can vary between 200 and 4000 mL. It is not indicated in all patients with OHSS, but is indicated in the following situations, which are guided by the symptoms of the patient [33].

- Significant abdominal distension and abdominal pain secondary to ascites.
- Shortness of breath and respiratory compromise secondary to ascites and increased intra-abdominal pressure.
- Oliguria despite adequate volume replacement, secondary to increased abdominal pressure, causing reduced renal perfusion.

After paracentesis, there is a significant decrease in the intra-abdominal pressure (IAP) with improved venous return and renal and uterine perfusion [34]. Repeat paracentesis may be indicated in those patients who become symptomatic again. Placement of an indwelling transabdominal pigtail catheter instead of repeated multiple paracentesis for continuous drainage of ascites in patients with OHSS can be an option [35]. The placement of a pigtail catheter is a safe and effective treatment modality for the management of ascites in severe OHSS [36].

Hydrothorax may accompany ascites and may require drainage in patients with severe dyspnoea and hypoxia in patients with severe OHSS [37]. Pericardial effusion, though rare, may occur in severe OHSS and requires drainage by an expert physician. [37].

Surgical Treatment Surgical treatment may be necessary for ruptured cysts or ovarian torsion. The surgery should be done preferably laparoscopically by a skilled surgeon so that oophorectomy can be avoided [38].

An alternative hCG protocol or lower dose of hCG used for the trigger, aspirin, cycle cancellation, dual trigger, elective single embryo transfer (e-SET) and use of Follitropin delta, inositol, insulin-sensitizing drugs, ketoconazole, Kisspeptin, luteal GnRH antagonist administration, and vitamin D do not have any evidence to be used in the management of OHSS.

12.5 Conclusion

OHSS is associated with substantial physical and psychosocial morbidity. To prevent OHSS, one should identify women at risk of high response before stimulation, based on outcome from a previous cycle, ovarian reserve markers (AFC and AMH) and age, which can predict ovarian response and occurrence of OHSS. In some women, OHSS is diagnosed after ovarian stimulation has been started. In these women with unexpected OHSS, one must adopt certain treatment strategies that aim at decreasing the severity of OHSS. Only a few interventions today can be considered effective in reducing the incidence of OHSS and its severity with high or moderate certainty of evidence in unexpected OHSS. Calcium, HES, and cabergoline are safe and effective in preventing moderate-to-severe OHSS. Apart from this, management should involve circulatory support using IV fluids, maintenance of renal function, thromboprophylaxis, and drainage of third-space accumulation if necessary. In severe OHSS, multidisciplinary management protocols involving gynaecologists, anaesthetists, and haematologists should be generated and strictly followed.

Compliance with guidelines and evidence-based best practices is essential for medicolegal purposes, especially in critical cases, as there are chances of morbidity and mortality. Effective care for unexpected OHSS begins with early diagnosis and identifying comorbidities and complications early to provide effective care. Psychological support for these patients is very important.

References

1. Jahromi BN, Parsanezhad ME, Shomali Z, Bakhshai P, Alborzi M, Vaziri NM, Anvar Z. Ovarian hyperstimulation syndrome: a narrative review of its pathophysiology, risk factors, prevention, classification, and management. Iranian journal of medical sciences. 2018;43(3):248.
2. Li HW, Lee VC, Lau EY, Yeung WS, Ho PC, Ng EH. Cumulative live-birth rate in women with polycystic ovary syndrome or isolated polycystic ovaries undergoing in-vitro fertilisation treatment. J Assist Reprod Genet. 2014;31:205–11.
3. Gullo G, Cucinella G, Stojanovic V, Stojkovic M, Bruno C, Streva AV, Lopez A, Perino A, Marinelli S. Ovarian Hyperstimulation syndrome (OHSS): a narrative review and legal implications. Journal of Personalized Medicine. 2024;14(9):91.
4. Nahid S, Alansari L, Ummunnisa F, Amara UE, Ramireddy N, Almarzooqi T. Ovarian hyperstimulation syndrome. In: Updates in intensive care of OBGY patients, vol. 24. Singapore: Springer; 2024. p. 181–208.
5. Rahimianfar F, Rahimianfar M, Eshghjoo S. The varied impacts of vascular endothelial growth factor-a (VEGF-a) on vasculature in ovarian hyper stimulation syndrome (OHSS) and obesity. Preprints: Preprints; 2023.
6. Fang L, Yu Y, Li Y, Wang S, He J, Zhang R, Sun YP. Upregulation of AREG, EGFR, and HER2 contributes to increased VEGF expression in granulosa cells of patients with OHSS. Biol Reprod. 2019;101(2):426–32.
7. Papanikolaou EG, Humaidan P, Polyzos N, Kalantaridou S, Kol S, Benadiva C, Tournaye H, Tarlatzis B. New algorithm for OHSS prevention. Reprod Biol Endocrinol. 2011;9:1–5.
8. Bosch E, Broer S, Griesinger G, Grynberg M, Humaidan P, Kolibianakis E, et al. ESHRE guideline: ovarian stimulation for IVF/ICSI. Human Reprod Open 2020;2.
9. ASRM. Practice Committee of the American society for reproductive medicine. Fertil Steril. 2016;106:1634e47.
10. Sun B, Ma Y, Li L, Hu L, Wang F, Zhang Y, et al. Factors associated with ovarian hyperstimulation syndrome (OHSS) severity in women with polycystic ovary syndrome undergoing IVF/ICSI. Front Endocrinol. 2020;11:615957.
11. Polyzos N, Neves A, Drakopoulos P, Spits C, Alvaro Mercadal B, Garcia S, et al. The effect of polymorphisms in FSHR and FSHB genes on ovarian response: a prospective multicenter multinational study in Europe and Asia. Hum Reprod. 2021;36:1711e21.

12. D'Angelo A, Amso NN, Hassan R. Coasting (withholding gonadotrophins) for preventing ovarian hyperstimulation syndrome. Cochrane Database Syst Rev 2017;5.
13. Mourad S, Brown J, Farquhar C. Interventions for the prevention of OHSS in ART cycles: an overview of Cochrane reviews. Cochrane Database Syst Rev 2017;1.
14. Kwan I, Bhattacharya S, Woolner A. Monitoring of stimulated cycles in assisted reproduction (IVF and ICSI). Cochrane Database Syst Rev. 2021;4:CD005289.
15. Fatemi H, Bilger W, Denis D, Griesinger G, La Marca A, Longobardi S, et al. Dose adjustment of follicle-stimulating hor-mone (FSH) during ovarian stimulation as part of medically-assisted reproduction in clinical studies: a systematic review covering 10 years (2007e2017). Reprod Biol Endocrinol. 2021;19:68.
16. Mahony M, Hayward B, Mottla G, Richter K, Beall S, Ball D, et al. Recombinant human follicle stimulating hormone alfa dose adjustment in US clinical practice: an observational, retrospective analysis of a real-world electronic medical records database. Front Endocrinol. 2021;12:1660.
17. Lensen S, Wilkinson J, Leijdekkers J, La Marca A, Mol B, Marjoribanks J, et al. Individualised gonadotropin dose selection using markers of ovarian reserve for women undergoing in vitro fertilisation plus intracytoplasmic sperm injection (IVF/ICSI). Cochrane Database Syst Rev. 2018;2:CD012693.
18. Youssef M, Van der Veen F, Al-Inany H, Mochtar M, Griesinger G, Nagi Mohesen M, et al. Gonadotropin-releasing hor-mone agonist versus HCG for oocyte triggering in antagonist-assisted reproductive technology (review). Cochrane Database Syst Rev. 2014;50:CD008046.
19. Papanikolaou EG, Verpoest W, Fatemi H, Tarlatzis B, Devroey P, Tournaye H. A novel method of luteal supplementation with recombinant luteinizing hormone when a gonadotropin-releasing hormone agonist is used instead of human chorionic gonadotropin for ovulation triggering: a randomized prospective proof of concept study. Fertil Steril. 2011;95(3):1174–7.
20. Youssef MA, Abou-Setta AM, Lam WS. Recombinant versus urinary human chorionic gonadotrophin for final oocyte maturation triggering in IVF and ICSI cycles. Cochrane Database Syst Rev. 2016;4:CD003719.
21. Tang H, Mourad S, Wang A, Zhai SD, Hart R. Dopamine agonists for preventing ovarian hyperstimulation syndrome. Cochrane Database Syst Rev. 2021;4:CD008605.
22. Fouda UM, Elshaer HS, Youssef GG, Hanafy A, Mehrem WM, Youssef MA, Farouk M, Nabil H. Cabergoline versus calcium infusion in the prevention of ovarian Hyperstimulation syndrome: a randomised controlled study. J Obstet Gynaecol. 2022;42:122–6.

23. Baradwan S, AlJaroudi D, Agdi M, Hafedh B, Abduljabbar HH, Sabban H, Alzawawi N, Alsaad N, Alshahrani MS, Idriss A, et al. Calcium versus Cabergoline for prevention of ovarian Hyperstimulation syndrome: a systematic review and meta-analysis. Eur J Obs Gynecol Reprod Biol. 2024;301:1–11.
24. Lotfalizadeh M, Khadem N, Sadeghi T, Jahanpak N, Mahmoudinia M, Faraji P, Zakerinasab F, Mahmoudinia M. The effect of intravenous calcium gluconate on the prevention of ovarian hyperstimulation syndrome. (a randomized clinical trial). Journal of gynecology obstetrics and human. Reproduction. 2024;53(10):102850.
25. Li T, Zhu W, Liu G, Fang C, Quan S. Diosmin for the prevention of ovarian hyperstimulation syndrome. Int J Gynecol Obstet. 2020 May;149(2):166–70.
26. Youssef MA, Mourad S. Volume expanders for the prevention of ovarian Hyperstimulation syndrome. Cochrane Database Syst Rev. 2016;2016:CD001302.
27. Wu D, Shi H, Yu Y, Yu T, Zhai J. Comparison of the effectiveness of various medicines in the prevention of ovarian hyperstimulation syndrome: a network meta-analysis of randomized controlled trials. Front Endocrinol. 2022;13:808517.
28. Sood A, Mathur R. Ovarian hyperstimulation syndrome. Obst Gynaecol Reprod Med. 2020;30(8):251–5.
29. Medwin C, Rozen G, Agresta F, Nassar N, Polyakov A. The ovarian hyperstimulation that truly matters: admissions, severity and prevention strategies. Aust N Z J Obstet Gynaecol. 2023;63(4):583–7.
30. Mor YS, Schenker JG. Ovarian hyperstimulation syndrome and thrombotic events. Am J Reprod Immunol. 2014;72(6):541–8.
31. Wormer KC, Jangda AA, El Sayed FA, Stewart KI, Mumford SL, Segars JH. Is thromboprophylaxis cost effective in ovarian hyperstimulation syndrome: a systematic review and cost analysis. Eur J Obstet Gynecol Reprod Biol. 2018;224:117–24.
32. Smith LP, Hacker MR, Alper MM. Patients with severe ovarian hyperstimulation syndrome can be managed safely with aggressive outpatient transvaginal paracentesis. Fertil Steril. 2009;92(6):1953–9.
33. Gebril A, Hamoda H, Mathur R. Outpatient management of severe ovarian hyperstimulation syndrome: a systematic review and a review of existing guidelines. Hum Fertil. 2018;21(2):98–105.
34. Levin I, Almog B, Avni A, Baram A, Lessing JB, Gamzu R. Effect of paracentesis of ascitic fluids on urinary output and blood indices in patients with severe ovarian hyperstimulation syndrome. Fertil Steril. 2002;77(5):986–8.
35. Dawood AS, Elsharwy MA. Continuous versus intermittent paracentesis in severe ovarian hyperstimulation syndrome: a multicenter randomized clinical trial. J Reprod Biol Endocrinol. 2017;1:23–8.

36. Abuzeid M, Warda H, Joseph S, Corrado MG, Abuzeid Y, Ashraf M, Rizk B. Outpatient management of severe ovarian hyperstimulation syndrome (OHSS) with placement of pigtail catheter. Facts Views Vis Obgyn. 2014;6(1):31.
37. Carter R, Petrie K, Sadighi A, Skene H. Ovarian hyperstimulation syndrome on the acute medical unit: a problem-based review. Acute Med. 2015;14(1):21–7.
38. Al Omari W, Ghazal-Aswad S, Sidky IH, Al Bassam MK. Ovarian salvage in bilaterally complicated severe ovarian hyperstimulation syndrome. Fertil Steril. 2011;96(2):e77–9.

Is HCG Trigger History?

13

Raoul Orvieto

13.1 Introduction

During the ovulatory cycle, estradiol production by the preovulatory follicle triggers the mid-cycle LH surge. This surge leads to various changes, including the separation of the oocyte from cumulus cells, cumulus expansion, germinal vesicle breakdown, meiosis resumption, and granulosa cell luteinization. Moreover, the subsequent rise in progesterone supports the positive feedback action of estradiol, inducing the midcycle FSH peak [1]. This peak FSH plays crucial roles, such as ensuring an adequate complement of LH receptors on the granulosa layer and synthesizing the hyaluronic acid matrix, enabling cumulus cell expansion. This allows the oocyte-cumulus cell mass to float freely in the antral [1].

R. Orvieto (✉)
Infertility and IVF Institute, Department of Obstetrics and Gynecology, Chaim Sheba Medical Center (Tel Hashomer), Ramat Gan, Israel

Tarnesby-Tarnowski Chair for Family Planning and Fertility Regulation, Gray Faculty of Medical and Health Science, Tel-Aviv University, Tel Aviv, Israel
e-mail: raoul.orvieto@sheba.health.gov.il

G. N. Allahbadia et al. (eds.), *Ovarian Hyperstimulation Syndrome (OHSS) Free Clinic*, https://doi.org/10.1007/978-981-95-3289-6_13

13.2 Human Chorionic Gonadotropin, a Surrogate to the Naturally Occurring LH Surge

In conventional controlled ovarian hyperstimulation (COH), final follicular maturation is typically triggered by a single dose of human chorionic gonadotropin (hCG) (5000–10,000 units), administered as close as possible to the time of ovulation (i.e., 36 h before oocyte recovery) [2]. Acting as a surrogate to the natural LH surge, hCG induces granulosa cell luteinization, final oocyte maturation, and resumption of meiosis.

Ovarian hyperstimulation syndrome (OHSS) almost always occurs either 3–7 days after hCG administration in susceptible patients (early onset) or during early pregnancy, 12–17 days after hCG administration (late onset). Individualization of treatment according to the specific risk factor and the specific response in the current cycle, with the option of freezing all embryos or replacing a single embryo, may mitigate the risk and severity of OHSS in susceptible cases [3]. Moreover, while withholding the ovulation-inducing trigger of hCG may eliminate severe early OHSS, it is associated with patient frustration and increased resource consumption.

13.3 Patients at Risk of Developing Severe OHSS

Controlled ovarian hyperstimulation, incorporating GnRH antagonist co-treatment and GnRH agonist (GnRHa) trigger, has emerged as a common approach to mitigate the risk of severe early OHSS and promote the concept of an OHSS-free clinic [4, 5]. However, concerns about reduced clinical pregnancy rates and increased first-trimester pregnancy loss [6, 7], have prompted exploration of alternative strategies to enhance reproductive outcomes. The following approaches have been proposed to address these concerns: freeze-all policy; fresh transfer and intensive luteal support; and fresh transfer with one bolus of 1500 IU hCG 1 h after oocyte retrieval [8–10]. While the latter was demonstrated to rescue the luteal phase, resulting in a reproductive outcome comparable with that of HCG triggering, when applied to patients at high risk of developing severe OHSS, 26% developed severe early OHSS requiring ascites drainage and hospitalization [11]. This figure is comparable to the acceptable 20% prevalence of severe OHSS in ostensibly high-risk patients [12].

Another suggested option is administering a single bolus of 1500 IU hCG 5 days after the initial GnRHa trigger, particularly for patients producing fewer than 20 oocytes [3, 13]. Following oocyte retrieval, patients start intensive luteal support and are evaluated for early signs of moderate OHSS. If no signs are detected, one embryo is transferred, and patients subsequently receive the delayed hCG bolus. This delayed approach, deferring hCG administration by 3 days, has shown promise in rescuing the corpus luteum, resulting in high midluteal progesterone levels, reasonable pregnancy rates, and no instances of severe OHSS [13]. However, the need for further large prospective randomized studies is emphasized due to the limited sample size of the preliminary results [13].

13.4 hCG Versus GnRHa Trigger

In the comparison of hCG and GnRHa triggers in the context of follicular maturation during IVF treatment cycles, studies have consistently shown that the GnRHa trigger yields comparable or even superior outcomes in key variables such as the number of retrieved oocytes, the percentage of mature oocytes, and the quantity of top-quality embryos, suggesting that the use of GnRHa as a trigger is associated with favorable results in terms of oocyte quality and developmental potential. Further insights into the downstream effects of LH receptor activation by LH or hCG reveal distinct pathways. LH has a more pronounced impact on AKT and extracellular signal-regulated protein kinase (ERK1/2) phosphorylation, processes crucial for granulosa cell proliferation, differentiation, and survival. On the other hand, hCG induces higher intracellular cAMP accumulation, stimulating steroidogenesis, particularly the production of progesterone [14]. Using similar design, Yung et al. [15] investigated the messenger RNA expression of reproduction-related genes in human GCs exposed to hCG; FSH and LH; or hCG, FSH, and LH. The exposure to LH + FSH + hCG showed higher activation of steroidogenesis (StAR/CYP19) and maturation (COX2/Amphiregulin)-related genes, as compared to the naturally occurring trigger (LH + FSH) and the hCG triggers. Moreover, while the naturally occurring trigger (LH + FSH) activated maturation significantly and more intensely than the hCG trigger, no in between group differences were observed with regard to steroidogenic-related genes.

Following the aforementioned findings, the combination of GnRHa with hCG for final follicular maturation has been integrated into clinical practice. It is emphasized that the various modes and timings of administration should be tailored to specific subgroups of IVF patients, acknowledging the diverse responses and characteristics within the patient population. This personalized approach aims to optimize the effectiveness of the trigger regimen in different clinical scenarios during assisted reproductive techniques.

13.5 Patients Not at Risk of Developing Severe OHSS

The aforementioned observations demonstrating a comparable or even better oocyte/embryos maturity and quality following GnRHa trigger, as compared to hCG trigger, along with the distinct effects of LH and hCG on downstream signaling through the LH receptor, have paved the way for a novel strategy in final follicular maturation. This involves the simultaneous administration of both GnRHa and a standard bolus of hCG (5000–10,000 units) before oocyte retrieval, aiming to enhance oocyte and embryo quality, thereby improving the overall outcome of IVF cycles.

13.5.1 Dual Trigger: Standard hCG Dose Concomitant with GnRHa, 35–37 H before Oocyte Retrieval

In a retrospective cohort study by Lin et al. [16], normal responder patients undergoing COH were compared based on the trigger protocol used. The study compared the outcomes of patients receiving a standard dosage of hCG trigger (6500 IU of rec hCG) versus a dual trigger (0.2 mg of triptorelin and 6500 IU of rec hCG) administered 35–36 h prior to oocyte retrieval. The dual trigger group exhibited a statistically significant higher number of retrieved oocytes, matured oocytes, and cryopreserved embryos, resulting in a significant increase in implantation rates, clinical pregnancy rates, and live-birth rates compared to the hCG-only trigger group.

In a subsequent prospective randomized controlled trial involving normal responder patients, Decleer et al. [17] compared the IVF outcomes following either a 5000 IU hCG trigger or a combination of GnRHa plus 5000 IU hCG administered concomitantly 36 h prior to oocyte retrieval. While no significant differences were observed between the groups in terms of the mean number of retrieved oocytes, matured oocytes, or pregnancy rates, the dual trigger group showed a significant advantage with respect to a higher number of patients in the dual trigger group who received at least one embryo of excellent quality, and there were more cryopreserved embryos in this group.

Haas et al. [18] randomized 155 normal responder patients to receive either hCG or a dual trigger for final oocyte maturation demonstrated that using a dual trigger for final follicular maturation resulted in improved outcomes. The use of a dual trigger significantly increased the number of oocytes retrieved, mature/metaphase-II (MII) oocytes, total number of blastocysts and top-quality blastocysts transferred compared with the hCG group. Moreover, the clinical pregnancy rate and the live birth rate per transfer were significantly higher in the dual trigger group compared with the hCG group [18].

13.5.2 Double Trigger: —GnRHa 40 h and Standard hCG Added 34 h Prior to OPU, Respectively

Beck-Fruchter et al. [19] presented a case involving recurrent empty follicle syndrome, successfully managed by a unique ovulation trigger approach. In this case, a “double trigger” was employed, involving the administration of GnRHa 40 h before oocyte retrieval, followed by the addition of hCG 34 h prior to the retrieval procedure. The authors hypothesized that extending the time between ovulation triggering and oocyte retrieval [20], combined with the GnRHa trigger inducing a simultaneous FSH surge, could overcome potential impairments in granulosa cell function, oocyte meiotic maturation, or cumulus expansion. This “double trigger” approach resulted in the successful aspiration of mature oocytes, leading to a subsequent pregnancy and delivery.

Inspired by these promising observations, the double trigger approach was offered to two groups of patients exhibiting abnormal final follicular maturation despite a normal response to COH. The first group consisted of patients with a low (<50%) number of oocytes retrieved relative to the number of dominant follicles (>14 mm in diameter) on the day of hCG administration [21]. The second group included patients with a low proportion of mature/metaphase-II (MII) oocytes (<66%) per the number of oocytes retrieved [22].

In both subgroups, the implementation of the double trigger resulted in significantly improved embryological variables, including the number of retrieved oocytes, MII oocytes, 2PN embryos, and top-quality embryos, compared to cycles using the hCG-only trigger. Moreover, these improvements were associated with acceptable pregnancy rates, suggesting the potential efficacy of the double trigger approach in addressing specific challenges related to final follicular maturation in these patient subgroups.

13.5.3 Dual/Double Trigger in Poor Ovarian Responders

In poor ovarian response (POR) patients, a significant concern often overlooked is the high incidence of premature luteinization/ovulation [23, 24]. To address this issue, early triggering of final follicular maturation is recommended when approaching a follicular size of 15–16 mm or by shortening the duration between the trigger and OPU, aiming to mitigate premature luteinization/ovulation. However, since shortening the interval between hCG priming and oocyte retrieval may decrease the percentage of mature oocytes [20], an additional measure to improve the number of oocytes retrieved to the number of follicles >10 mm, and the proportion of mature oocytes should be implemented [21, 22]. In cases where, at the end of stimulation, the follicles measure >17 mm in diameter, or < 17 mm, specific strategies are recommended:

For follicles >17 mm: Consider a dual trigger administered 34 h prior to OPU to prevent premature ovulation and ensure the retrieval of a cohort of mature oocytes.

For follicles <17 mm: Implement a double trigger to achieve the same goal, addressing the specific needs of these smaller follicles.

These tailored approaches aim to optimize oocyte retrieval in POR patients by balancing the challenges associated with premature luteinization/ovulation and the need for mature oocytes.

13.6 Conclusions

In this chapter, we have conducted an analysis and discussion of the studies published to date, focusing on the various modes of combining GnRH agonist (GnRHa) with hCG trigger for final follicular maturation. The goal is to provide insights into how each mode can be tailored to suit specific individual patient characteristics and responses (see Fig. 13.1).

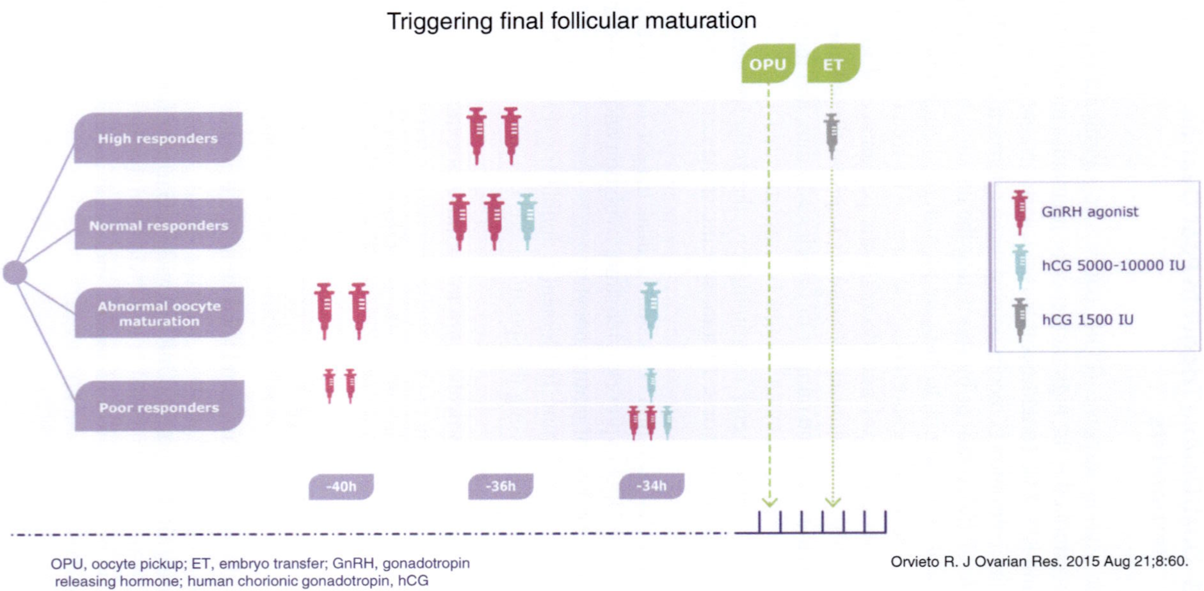

Fig. 13.1 The different modes of triggering ovulation

The researches discussed in this chapter encompass diverse trigger strategies, including GnRHa trigger alone, hCG trigger alone, and the combination of both triggers. By exploring the outcomes of these different trigger approaches, we seek to understand how they can be customized to address the unique needs and profiles of specific patient subgroups undergoing assisted reproductive techniques. The ultimate aim is to contribute to the refinement of trigger protocols, promoting personalized and effective approaches to final follicular maturation in the context of COH for IVF.

References

1. Fritz MA, Speroff L. Regulation of the menstrual cycle. In: Clinical gynecologic endocrinology and infertility. 8th ed. Philadelphia: Lippincott Williams & Wilkins; 2011.
2. Ludwig M, Doody KJ, Doody KM. Use of recombinant human chorionic gonadotropin in ovulation induction. Fertil Steril. 2003;79:1051–9.
3. Orvieto R. Ovarian hyperstimulation syndrome- an optimal solution for an unresolved enigma. J Ovarian Res. 2013;6:77.
4. Orvieto R. Can we eliminate severe ovarian hyperstimulation syndrome? Hum Reprod. 2005;20:320–2.
5. Devroey P, Polyzos NP, Blockeel C. An OHSS-free clinic by segmentation of IVF treatment. Hum Reprod. 2011;6:2593–7.
6. Youssef MA, Van der Veen F, Al-Inany HG, Mochtar MH, Griesinger G, Nagi Mohesen M, Aboulfoutouh I, van Wely M Gonadotropin-releasing hormone agonist versus HCG for oocyte triggering in antagonist-assisted reproductive technology.Cochrane Database Syst Rev 2014 31;(10):CD008046.
7. Orvieto R, Rabinson J, Meltzer S, Zohav E, Anteby E, Homburg R. Substituting HCG with GnRH agonist to trigger final follicular maturation–a retrospective comparison of three different ovarian stimulation protocols. Reprod Biomed Online. 2006;13:198–201.
8. Humaidan P, Bungum L, Bungum M, Yding AC. Rescue of corpus luteum function with peri-ovulatory HCG supplementation in IVF/ICSI GnRH antagonist cycles in which ovulation was triggered with a GnRH agonist: a pilot study. Reprod Biomed Online. 2006;13:173–8.
9. Humaidan P, Bredkjaer HE, Westergaard LG, Andersen CY. 1,500 IU human chorionic gonadotropin administered at oocyte retrieval rescues the luteal phase when gonadotropin- releasing hormone agonist is used for ovulation induction: a prospective, randomized, controlled study. Fertil Steril. 2010;93:847–54.

10. Humaidan P, Papanikolaou EG, Kyrou D, Alsbjerg B, Polyzos NP, Devroey P, Fatemi HM. The luteal phase after GnRH-agonist triggering of ovulation: present and future perspectives. Reprod Biomed Online. 2012;24:134–41.
11. Seyhan A, Ata B, Polat M, Son WY, Yarali H, Dahan MH. Severe early ovarian hyperstimulation syndrome following GnRH agonist trigger with the addition of 1500 IU hCG. Hum Reprod. 2013;28:2522–8.
12. Orvieto R, Ben-Rafael Z. Role of intravenous albumin in the prevention of severe ovarian hyperstimulation syndrome. Hum Reprod. 1998;13:3306–9.
13. Haas J, Kedem A, Machtinger R, Dar S, Hourovitz A, Yerushalmi G, Orvieto R. HCG (1500IU) administration on day 3 after oocytes retrieval, following GnRH-agonist trigger for final follicular maturation, results in high sufficient mid luteal progesterone levels – a proof of concept. J Ovarian Res. 2014;7:35.
14. Casarini L, Lispi M, Longobardi S, Milosa F, La Marca A, Tagliasacchi D, Pignatti E, Simoni M. LH and hCG action on the same receptor results in quantitatively and qualitatively different intracellular signalling. PLoS One. 2012;7:e46682.
15. Yung Y, Aizer A, Tieb S, Avhar Maydan S, Maman E, Marom Haham L, Haas J, Orvieto R. The in-vitro effect of gonadotropins' type and combination on granulosa cells gene expressions. Reprod Biol Endocrinol. 2022;20:144.
16. Lin MH, Wu FS, Lee RK, Li SH, Lin SY, Hwu YM. Dual trigger with combination of gonadotropin-releasing hormone agonist and human chorionic gonadotropin significantly improves the live-birth rate for normal responders in GnRH-antagonist cycles. Fertil Steril. 2013;100:1296–302.
17. Decleer W, Osmanagaoglu K, Seynhave B, Kolibianakis S, Tarlatzis B, Devroey P. Comparison of hCG triggering versus hCG in combination with a GnRH agonist: a prospective randomized controlled trial. Facts Views Vis Obgyn. 2014;6:203–9.
18. Haas J, Bassil R, Samara N, Zilberberg E, Mehta C, Orvieto R, et al. GnRH agonist and hCG (dual trigger) versus hCG trigger for final follicular maturation: a double-blinded. Randomized Controlled Stud Hum Reprod (Oxford England). 2020;35(7):1648–54.
19. Beck-Fruchter R, Weiss A, Lavee M, Geslevich Y, Shalev E. Empty follicle syndrome: successful treatment in a recurrent case and review of the literature. Hum Reprod. 2012;27:1357–67.
20. Wang W, Zhang XH, Wang WH, Liu YL, Zhao LH, Xue SL, Yang KH. The time interval between hCG priming and oocyte retrieval in ART program: a meta-analysis. J Assist Reprod Genet. 2011;28:901–10.
21. Haas J, Zilberberg E, Dar S, Kedem A, Machtinger R, Orvieto R. Co-administration of GnRH-agonist and hCG for final oocyte maturation (double trigger) in patients with low number of oocytes retrieved per

number of preovulatory follicles-a preliminary report. J Ovarian Res. 2014;7:77.

22. Zilberberg E, Haas J, Dar S, Kedem A, Machtinger R, Orvieto R. Co-administration of GnRH-agonist and hCG for final oocyte maturation in patients with low proportion of mature oocytes. Gynecol Endocrinol. 2015;31:145–7.
23. Martinez F, Barri PN, Coroleu B, Tur R, Sorsa-Leslie T, Harris WJ, Groome NP, Knight PG, Fowler PA. Women with poor response to IVF have lowered circulating gonadotrophin surge-attenuating factor (GnSAF) bioactivity during spontaneous and stimulated cycles. Hum Reprod. 2002;17:634–40.
24. Ben-Rafael Z, Orvieto R, Feldberg D. The poor-responder patient in an in-vitro fertilization-embryo transfer (IVF-ET) program. Gynecol Endocrinol. 1994;8:277–86.

The Role of Ultrasound in Minimizing Morbidity in OHSS

14

Yenon Hazan, Inbal Navon, and Sharon Perlman

14.1 Introduction

Ovarian hyperstimulation syndrome (OHSS) is the most severe iatrogenic complication of ovarian stimulation in assisted reproductive technology (ART) procedures.

Y. Hazan (✉)
Department of Obstetrics and Gynecology, Kaplan Medical Center, Rehovot, Israel

The Hebrew University and Hadassah Medical School, Jerusalem, Israel
e-mail: pochy@netvision.net.il

I. Navon
The Helen Schneider Women's Hospital, Rabin Medical Center, Petach-Tikva, Israel

Gray Faculty of Medical and Health Sciences, Tel Aviv University, Tel Aviv, Israel

S. Perlman
Gray Faculty of Medical and Health Sciences, Tel Aviv University, Tel Aviv, Israel

Liss Maternity and Womens Hospital, Tel Aviv Sourasky Medical Center, Tel Aviv, Israel

G. N. Allahbadia et al. (eds.), *Ovarian Hyperstimulation Syndrome (OHSS) Free Clinic*, https://doi.org/10.1007/978-981-95-3289-6_14

While the pathophysiology of OHSS is not fully understood, its hallmark features include capillary leak and third spacing. These factors can lead to hemoconcentration, thromboembolic complications, fluid balance disturbances, ascites, pleural and pericardial effusions, and can even be fatal. Based on clinical, laboratory, and imaging findings, the severity of OHSS is classified as mild to critical. Moderate-to-severe cases of OHSS account for 3–5% of all ART treatments, as documented in national surveys [1–2].

Extensive research supports various strategies to prevent or lessen the occurrence of moderate-to-severe OHSS cases.

Preventing severe OHSS is the cornerstone of effective management, and vigilant monitoring throughout the stimulation protocol significantly reduces this risk. The key to primary prevention involves identifying high-risk individuals and tailoring treatment protocols accordingly. Strategies include administering dopamine agonists to high-risk patients and metformin to those with polycystic ovary syndrome (PCOS) [3]. Additionally, employing a GnRH antagonist protocol with GnRH-agonist triggering for hyperresponsive patients or opting for cryopreservation of all embryos (freeze-all) instead of immediate fresh embryo transfer is also essential.

Even after the diagnosis of OHSS is made, timely interventions can reduce OHSS-related morbidity and mortality. Despite extensive efforts to lower the incidence of OHSS, it remains a significant health concern in ART and a considerable financial burden. In this chapter, we review the role of ultrasound imaging and ultrasound-guided procedures in lowering OHSS-related morbidity.

14.2 The Role of Ultrasound in Fertility Treatments

Ultrasound imaging plays a crucial role in fertility treatments. Monitoring ovarian response in these treatments mainly involves pelvic ultrasound and blood tests to assess estradiol, progesterone, and LH levels.

Kwan's Cochrane review from 2021 [4] suggested that incorporating blood tests alongside transvaginal ultrasound (TVUS) does not yield better outcomes or reduce the risk of OHSS. While frequent testing can be time-consuming, costly, and inconvenient for patients, there remains a belief that continuous monitoring, which includes both TVUS and serum estradiol concentrations, is upheld by some as the gold standard for managing stimulation cycles to optimize follicle development, timing of embryo transfer, and mitigating the risks of OHSS.

The debate continues over the optimal level of monitoring, as it can lead to adjustments in treatment, such as modifying gonadotropin doses to prevent OHSS and other complications.

14.3 The Role of Ultrasound in the Detection and Management of OHSS

Ultrasound is a noninvasive and effective method for identifying high-risk factors, continuously monitoring, and detecting early signs of OHSS development.

14.3.1 Risk Assessment Prior to Treatment: Baseline Characteristics

Identifying high-risk patients is the first step in the primary prevention of OHSS, as it allows for proper precautions in terms of the stimulation protocol and the selection of treatment parameters. Known risk factors for OHSS include PCOS, young age, previous OHSS, high antral follicular count (AFC), low BMI, and elevated anti-Müllerian hormone (AMH) levels.

Among these risk factors, TVUS is particularly effective for diagnosing polycystic ovary syndrome (PCOS) and detecting a high antral follicle count (AFC) of more than 24 small antral follicles. PCOS is the most common endocrine disorder affecting women of reproductive age. The diagnosis of polycystic ovary syndrome is based on the modified 2003 Rotterdam criteria, which include clinical, biochemical, and sonographic. The sonographic criteria involve having 20 or more follicles in either ovary or an ovarian volume of at least 10 cm^3, measured using a transvaginal transducer with a frequency of 8 MHz or higher [5].

14.3.2 Risk Assessment During Treatment

The development of multiple follicles in response to gonadotropin stimulation independently predicts the risk of OHSS. The threshold typically ranges from 20 to 24 follicles measuring over 14 mm, with estradiol levels exceeding 3500 pg/mL.

US findings indicating pending OHSS include the number and size of the follicles, ovarian volume and diameter, the location and position of the ovaries (abdominal, "kissing ovaries"), and the presence of ascites. Integrating these ultrasound findings with clinical data offers valuable insights for adjusting treatment protocols and preventing OHSS.

As the number and size of follicles significantly impact the risk assessment for OHSS, research efforts have focused on the feasibility, applicability, and clinical yield of advanced ultrasound technologies that automatically count and measure ovarian follicle width and volume using various 3D software (Figs. 14.1 and 14.2). Promising potential benefits include reduced examination time for operators and patients, improved data storage capabilities, offline reconstruction options, and decreased inter- and intraobserver variability. However, studies validating the clinical efficacy and effects on fertility outcomes after implementing such technologies, compared to standard conventional monitoring of IVF treatments that use follicular diameter, are still pending [6–8].

Increased blood flow and AFC, which are significant risk factors for OHSS, characterize the ovaries in PCOS. Consequently, research has focused on the utility of ovarian vessel Doppler flow indices in predicting OHSS [9]. Although early studies [10, 11] demonstrated changes in Doppler blood flow velocities in the ovarian and uterine blood vessels of women with OHSS, later reports [9, 12, 13] utilizing three-dimensional power Doppler did not consistently show increased ovarian blood flow or other associated Doppler indices with OHSS. It appears that color Doppler

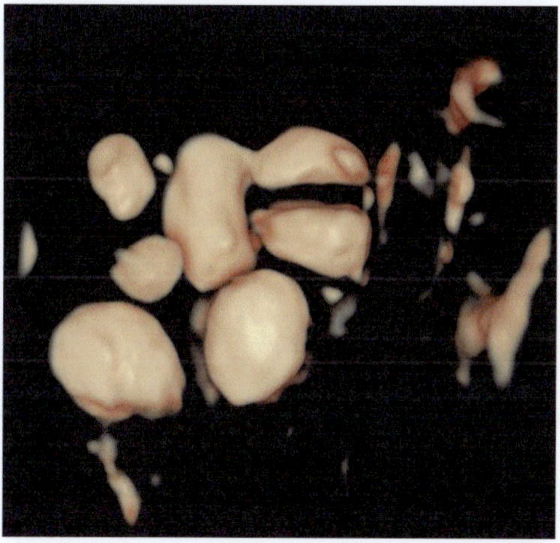

Fig. 14.1 A three-dimensional rendering inversion mode transvaginal ultrasound image of the ovary, obtained from a patient with OHSS, demonstrating multiple follicles. Measurement of the dimensions and volume of the follicles can be performed offline

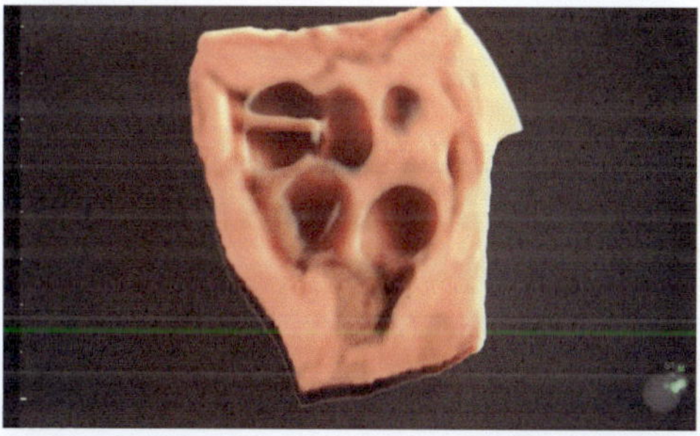

Fig. 14.2 Three-dimensional render mode transvaginal ultrasound image of an ovary from a patient referred for antral follicular count before IVF treatment

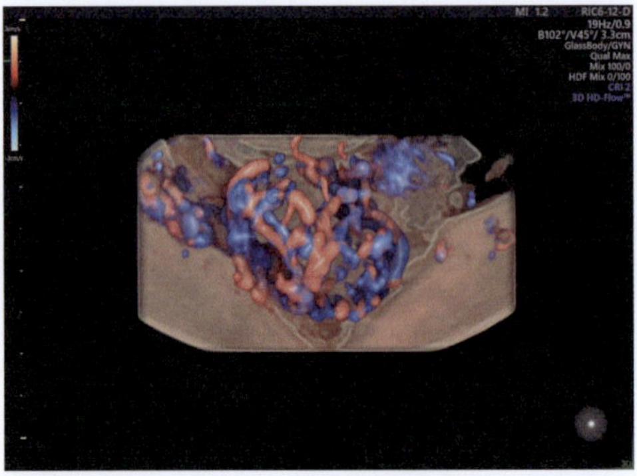

Fig. 14.3 Transvaginal image, using three-dimensional power Doppler angiography, demonstrating ovarian blood flow

and power Doppler need to be standardized and performed under identical conditions; thus, these methods are primarily useful for comparing changes over time within the same patient rather than for predicting OHSS (Fig. 14.3). Based on the current literature, circulatory changes linked to PCOS or fertility treatments cannot predict the onset of OHSS.

14.4 Ultrasound Applications for Severe OHSS Complications

Symptoms of OHSS are often nonspecific. Abdominal discomfort and shortness of breath are common; however, they may indicate severe, potentially life-threatening complications of OHSS, such as ascites, pleural effusion, and deep vein thrombosis, which highlight the importance of ultrasound in the diagnostic process [14, 15].

Ultrasonography is regarded as the primary method for investigating ART complications, particularly for the early detection and management of issues related to OHSS, as well as for guiding therapeutic interventions that can be applied across various clinical settings.

When compared to other diagnostic tools like CT scans or MRIs, ultrasound is cost-effective, making it the preferred choice for evaluating and treating OHSS.

14.4.1 Ultrasound-Guided Interventions for Severe OHSS

Ultrasonography is the first-line imaging modality for evaluating complications of OHSS. US-guided interventions for pleural effusion and ascites provide diagnostic insights and critical symptomatic relief [15, 16].

Ultrasound-guided thoracentesis is performed for pleural effusions that cause respiratory distress. To ensure safe needle insertion, ultrasound imaging accurately locates the fluid, which is then aspirated to relieve symptoms. The patient typically sits on the edge of a bed or chair, leaning forward on a table. Prior to the procedure, an ultrasound is conducted to determine the location of the fluid accumulation. Ultrasound accurately maps the area to guide needle insertion, reducing the risk of injury to the lungs or other structures in the chest. Afterward, the skin on the chest area where the needle will be inserted is cleaned and sterilized. A needle or catheter is carefully inserted into the pleural space, guided by ultrasound imaging, and fluid is withdrawn. Patients should experience immediate relief of symptoms following the procedure. After the procedure, a follow-up ultrasound or chest X-ray may be performed to ensure that the fluid has been adequately removed and to check for any potential complications, such as pneumothorax (Fig. 14.4). Utilizing ultrasound significantly reduces the risks associated with the procedure (bleeding, pneumothorax, and injury to the liver or spleen) by providing real-time imaging that helps avoid injury to nearby structures.

Ascites frequently leads to abdominal discomfort and respiratory difficulties, which may be alleviated by ultrasound-guided paracentesis (Fig. 14.5). The patient is usually instructed to lie on their back. Before the procedure, an ultrasound scan is carried out to locate the fluid in the abdominal cavity and to identify the safest site for needle insertion, typically on the left side of the

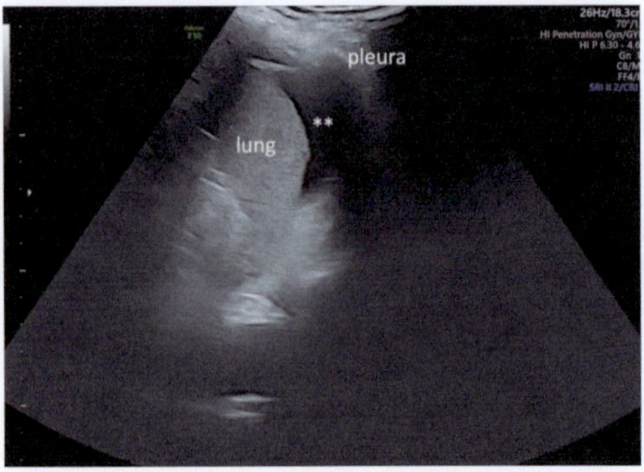

Fig. 14.4 An ultrasound image obtained from a patient with severe OHSS presenting with shortness of breath demonstrates the lung, the pleura, and the accumulation of fluid within the pleural space (**)

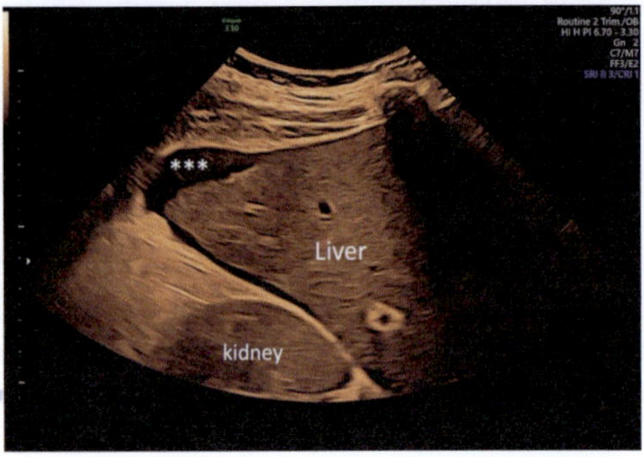

Fig. 14.5 An ultrasound image of the right upper abdominal quadrant obtained from a patient with severe OHSS presenting with abdominal discomfort, demonstrating fluid accumulation (***) between the liver and the kidney

patient, to avoid the liver. Care should be taken to prevent injury to the bowel, which may be distended due to ascites accumulation. Local anesthesia may be administered to minimize discomfort during the procedure. A needle, either attached to a syringe or a catheter connected to a vacuum bottle, is inserted through the skin and into the abdominal cavity, guided by ultrasound imaging. The fluid is then aspirated under direct visualization to ensure satisfactory fluid removal. Transvaginal drainage is also applicable and preferred by some practitioners. Immediate relief of abdominal and respiratory discomfort should follow the procedure.

Both procedures can be done at the bedside and carry minimal risks when conducted with ultrasound guidance.

14.4.2 Diagnosing Deep Vein Thrombosis (DVT)

OHSS can be associated with both arterial and venous thrombotic complications. These events (especially venous thrombosis) have also been reported to occur weeks after OHSS has resolved, and they can present in unusual sites (upper extremities), resulting in diagnostic and treatment challenges [17].

Ultrasound (US) is a noninvasive and highly effective technique for visualizing blood flow and identifying deep vein thrombosis (DVT) in the lower extremities. The primary method for detecting DVT via ultrasound is duplex ultrasound, which combines traditional ultrasound imaging with Doppler ultrasound. This dual approach assesses venous blood flow, identifying obstructions indicative of a clot, such as a segment of a vein showing no blood flow, direct visualization of a clot, or a vein that remains uncompressed under probe pressure. This method offers numerous advantages, including its noninvasive nature, avoidance of ionizing radiation exposure, feasibility for bedside or outpatient use, and high accuracy in identifying DVT, particularly in proximal veins. However, it may have limitations in detecting clots in calf veins or in individuals with a high body mass index (BMI) [18]. Ultrasound is also valuable for diagnosing upper extremity and jugular vein thrombosis, as well as the rare cases of ovarian vein thrombosis associated with assisted reproductive technology (ART) and ovarian hyperstimulation syndrome (OHSS). In such instances, an echocardiogram should be performed to assess whether the clot has extended to the vena cava and the heart [19].

14.4.3 Ultrasound Diagnosis of Ovarian Torsion

OHSS is characterized by two factors that increase the risk for ovarian torsion: the first, enlarged ovaries with a different center of mass, which are prone to twisting on their ligaments; the second, fluid accumulation within the abdomen, increases the potential for ovarian mobility, further increasing the risk for ovarian torsion and ovarian ischemia.

Complaints and imaging findings related to OHSS can resemble ovarian torsion. Specifically, abdominal pain often occurs due to an enlarged ovary and the build-up of free fluid in the abdominal cavity, alongside nausea and vomiting. Likewise, commonly observed imaging findings, like an enlarged ovary and free fluid, are less significant in this context.

Key ultrasound indicators of ovarian torsion in a patient with OHSS include diffuse ovarian edema, with follicles displaced to the periphery, reduced or absent blood flow in the affected ovary on color Doppler imaging (noting that normal blood flow does not necessarily rule out torsion), and the whirlpool sign, indicating a twisted vascular pedicle and strongly suggesting torsion [20].

A high index of suspicion, prompt diagnosis, and immediate intervention are crucial to prevent prolonged irreversible ovarian ischemia and rare complications such as ovarian autoamputation. It should be noted that the risk for ovarian torsion decreases; however, it does not diminish when the OHSS has resolved.

14.5 Advancements in Ovarian Stimulation Monitoring and OHSS Diagnosis

14.5.1 Point of Care Ultrasound

Point-of-care ultrasonography (POCUS) is a portable bedside ultrasound used for rapid diagnostics, particularly in emergency medicine. It is more sensitive and specific than a physical examination for conditions like ascites, pleural effusion, and pericardial effusion. POCUS can accurately detect free intraperitoneal fluid, even in the hands of inexperienced operators.

Moderate-to-severe cases of OHSS may present with nonspecific symptoms, including shortness of breath, abdominal bloating, nausea, and vomiting. POCUS has been documented in several case reports as a tool to aid and expedite the diagnosis of severe OHSS in emergency department settings, proving to be a valuable supplement to a focused history and physical examination. A more comprehensive implementation of POCUS will enhance the diagnosis and management of OHSS in outpatient settings [21, 22].

14.5.2 Future Innovations for Patient Self-Monitoring

Advancements in medical technology are reshaping the landscape of reproductive health, aiming to enhance patient empowerment and improve outcomes.

Innovations in monitoring ovarian stimulation aim to provide patients with greater autonomy and convenience in managing their fertility treatments. One potential advancement is a portable ultrasound device enhanced with user-friendly mobile guidance apps that offer real-time feedback and assistance, empowering patients to take an active role in their treatment process. Additionally, home-based hormone tests provide a noninvasive means for patients to monitor their hormonal profiles, facilitating personalized adjustments to stimulation protocols and minimizing the need for frequent clinic visits.

By leveraging these innovative ultrasound and other technologies, the monitoring of ovarian stimulation becomes more patient-centered, streamlined, and accessible, leading to better compliance and more accurate follow-up. Medical applications for mobile devices that aggregate patient data, including sonographic evaluations of the ovaries, have the potential to utilize AI algorithms for early detection of high-risk patients prone to developing OHSS, thereby alerting their physician promptly.

As the field continues to embrace patient empowerment and personalized care, the integration of innovative monitoring technologies signals a new era in fertility management, empowering patients to actively participate in their reproductive health journey.

References

1. Navot D, Bergh PA, Laufer N. Ovarian hyperstimulation syndrome in novel reproductive technologies: prevention and treatment. Fertil Steril. 1992;58(2):249–61. https://doi.org/10.1016/s0015-0282(16)55188-7. Erratum in: Fertil Steril 1993 Jun;59(6):1334. PMID: 1633889.
2. Kuroda K, Nagai S, Ikemoto Y, Matsumura Y, Ochiai A, Nojiri S, Itakura A, Sugiyama R. Incidences and risk factors of moderate-to-severe ovarian hyperstimulation syndrome and severe hemoperitoneum in 1,435,108 oocyte retrievals. Reprod Biomed Online. 2021;42(1):125–32. https://doi.org/10.1016/j.rbmo.2020.09.001. Epub 2020 Sep 3. PMID: 33051135.
3. Practice Committee of the American Society for Reproductive Medicine. Electronic address: ASRM@asrm.org; Practice Committee of the American Society for Reproductive Medicine. Prevention and treatment of moderate and severe ovarian hyperstimulation syndrome: a guideline. Fertil Steril. 2016;106(7):1634–47. https://doi.org/10.1016/j.fertnstert.2016.08.048. Epub 2016 Sep 24. PMID: 27678032.
4. Kwan I, Bhattacharya S, Woolner A. Monitoring of stimulated cycles in assisted reproduction (IVF and ICSI). Cochrane Database Syst Rev. 2021;4(4):CD005289. https://doi.org/10.1002/14651858.CD005289.pub4. PMID: 33844275; PMCID: PMC8094870.
5. Rotterdam ESHRE/ASRM-Sponsored PCOS Consensus Workshop Group. Revised 2003 consensus on diagnostic criteria and long-term health risks related to polycystic ovary syndrome. Fertil Steril. 2004;81(1):19–25. https://doi.org/10.1016/j.fertnstert.2003.10.004. PMID: 14711538.
6. Rodríguez-Fuentes A, Hernández J, García-Guzman R, Chinea E, Iaconianni L, Palumbo A. Prospective evaluation of automated follicle monitoring in 58 in vitro fertilization cycles: follicular volume as a new indicator of oocyte maturity. Fertil Steril. 2010;93(2):616–20. https://doi.org/10.1016/j.fertnstert.2009.02.058. Epub 2009 Apr 18. PMID: 19376513.
7. Peres Fagundes PA, Chapon R, Olsen PR, Schuster AK, Mattia MMC, Cunha-Filho JS. Evaluation of three-dimensional SonoAVC ultrasound for antral follicle count in infertile women: its agreement with conventional two-dimensional ultrasound and serum levels of anti-Müllerian

hormone. Reprod Biol Endocrinol. 2017;15(1):96. https://doi.org/10.1186/s12958-017-0314-x. PMID: 29246176; PMCID: PMC5732451.

8. Wertheimer A, Nagar R, Oron G, Meizner I, Fisch B, Ben-Haroush A. Fertility treatment outcomes after follicle tracking with standard 2-dimensional sonography versus 3-dimensional sonography-based automated volume count: prospective study. J Ultrasound Med. 2018;37(4):859–66. https://doi.org/10.1002/jum.14421. Epub 2017 Sep 29. PMID: 28960452.
9. Jayaprakasan K, Jayaprakasan R, Al-Hasie HA, Clewes JS, Campbell BK, Johnson IR, Raine-Fenning NJ. Can quantitative three-dimensional power Doppler angiography be used to predict ovarian hyperstimulation syndrome? Ultrasound Obstet Gynecol. 2009;33(5):583–91. https://doi.org/10.1002/uog.6373. Erratum in: Ultrasound Obstet Gynecol 2009 Oct;34(4):489. PMID: 19402100.
10. Agrawal R, Conway G, Sladkevicius P, Tan SL, Engmann L, Payne N, Bekir J, Campbell S, Jacobs H. Serum vascular endothelial growth factor and Doppler blood flow velocities in in vitro fertilization: relevance to ovarian hyperstimulation syndrome and polycystic ovaries. Fertil Steril. 1998;70(4):651–8. https://doi.org/10.1016/s0015-0282(98)00249-0. PMID: 9797093.
11. Tekay A, Martikainen H, Jouppila P. Doppler parameters of the ovarian and uterine blood circulation in ovarian hyperstimulation syndrome. Ultrasound Obstet Gynecol. 1995;6(1):50–3. https://doi.org/10.1046/j.1469-0705.1995.06010050.x. PMID: 8528802.
12. Mercé LT, Barco MJ, Bau S, Troyano JM. Prediction of ovarian response and IVF/ICSI outcome by three-dimensional ultrasonography and power Doppler angiography. Eur J Obstet Gynecol Reprod Biol. 2007;132(1):93–100. https://doi.org/10.1016/j.ejogrb.2006.07.051. Epub 2007 Feb 27. PMID: 17329008.
13. Pan HA, Wu MH, Cheng YC, Wu LH, Chang FM. Quantification of ovarian Doppler signal in hyperresponders during in vitro fertilization treatment using three-dimensional power Doppler ultrasonography. Ultrasound Med Biol. 2003;29(7):921–7. https://doi.org/10.1016/s0301-5629(03)00901-3. PMID: 12878236.
14. Selter J, Wen T, Palmerola KL, Friedman AM, Williams Z, Forman EJ. Life-threatening complications among women with severe ovarian hyperstimulation syndrome. Am J Obstet Gynecol. 2019;220(6):575.e1–575.e11. https://doi.org/10.1016/j.ajog.2019.02.009. Epub 2019 Feb 8. PMID: 30742828.
15. Ma X, Yin J, Yang R, Yang S, Li J, Wang Y, Li R. Clinical features of severe ovarian Hyperstimulation syndrome with hydrothorax. J Clin Med. 2023;12(19):6210. https://doi.org/10.3390/jcm12196210. PMID: 37834853; PMCID: PMC10573803.

16. Irani M, Robles A, Gunnala V, Chung P, Rosenwaks Z. Unilateral pleural effusion as the sole clinical presentation of severe ovarian hyperstimulation syndrome: a systematic review. Gynecol Endocrinol. 2018;34(2):92–9. https://doi.org/10.1080/09513590.2017.1390738. Epub 2017 Oct 24. Erratum in: Gynecol Endocrinol. 2018 Apr;34(4):ii. PMID: 29063807.
17. Needleman L, Cronan JJ, Lilly MP, Merli GJ, Adhikari S, Hertzberg BS, DeJong MR, Streiff MB, Meissner MH. Ultrasound for lower extremity deep venous thrombosis: multidisciplinary recommendations from the society of radiologists in ultrasound consensus conference. Circulation. 2018 137(14):1505-1515. Mor YS, Schenker JG. Ovarian hyperstimulation syndrome and thrombotic events. Am J Reprod Immunol 2014;72(6):541–8. https://doi.org/10.1111/aji.12310. Epub 2014 Aug 22. PMID: 25146913.
18. Chan WS, Ginsberg JS. A review of upper extremity deep vein thrombosis in pregnancy: unmasking the 'ART' behind the clot. J Thromb Haemost. 2006;4(8):1673–7. https://doi.org/10.1111/j.1538-7836.2006.02026.x. PMID: 16879207.
19. Berkkanoglu M, Coetzee K, Bulut H, Ozgur K. Risk of ovarian torsion is reduced in GnRH agonist triggered freeze-all cycles: a retrospective cohort study. J Obstet Gynaecol. 2019;39(2):212–7. https://doi.org/10.1080/01443615.2018.1479381. Epub 2018 Sep 19. PMID: 30230393.
20. Moro F, Bolomini G, Sibal M, Vijayaraghavan SB, Venkatesh P, Nardelli F, Pasciuto T, Mascilini F, Pozzati F, Leone FPG, Josefsson H, Epstein E, Guerriero S, Scambia G, Valentin L, Testa AC. Imaging in gynecological disease (20): clinical and ultrasound characteristics of adnexal torsion. Ultrasound Obstet Gynecol. 2020;56(6):934–43. https://doi.org/10.1002/uog.21981. Epub 2020 Nov 10. PMID: 31975482.
21. Osakwe E, Meighan V, Cunningham K, Morrissey B. Point of care ultrasound in the diagnosis and Management of Severe Ovarian Hyperstimulation Syndrome. Ir Med J. 2020;113(1):11. PMID: 32298563.
22. Bellapu S, Guttman J. Use of point-of-care ultrasound for the diagnosis of ovarian Hyperstimulation syndrome. J Emerg Med. 2017;52(4):e101–4. https://doi.org/10.1016/j.jemermed.2016.11.026. Epub 2016 Dec 18. PMID: 27998636.

15 Is In Vitro Maturation (IVM) Still Relevant for an OHSS-Free Clinic?

Shahar Kol

15.1 Rationale

Conventional IVF, as practiced for many years, relies on ovarian stimulation with gonadotropins, triggering final oocyte maturation, and retrieval of mature, metaphase II, oocytes to be fertilized in the IVF lab. This practice is not devoid of disadvantages: it involves the use of expensive medications (gonadotropins, GnRH analogs) administered by injections and potentially exposes the patient to the risk of OHSS. The rationale behind IVM is to eliminate these two disadvantages by retrieving immature oocytes from unstimulated antral follicles, followed by achieving fertilizable oocytes in vitro. In the context of OHSS, since no CL are created, OHSS is totally eliminated. Indeed, OHSS-high-risk patients (with high antral follicle count) are potential candidates for IVM.

S. Kol (✉)
IVF Unit, Bnai Zion Medical Center, Haifa, Israel
e-mail: kol@medica.co.il

G. N. Allahbadia et al. (eds.), *Ovarian Hyperstimulation Syndrome (OHSS) Free Clinic*, https://doi.org/10.1007/978-981-95-3289-6_15

15.2 Introduction

The idea and rationale of maturing human oocytes in vitro are old ones. The "father of IVF," the late Professor Robert Edwards, who was awarded the Nobel Prize in Physiology or Medicine in 2010, suggested this option in 1965 [1]. This technology is no longer considered experimental [2]; however, it never gained wide clinical acceptance and use, like other technologies in the field of ART, most notably, intracytoplasmic sperm injection (ICSI). The IVM technology is based on collecting immature oocytes from hormonally unstimulated, or minimally primed follicles, to be matured and fertilized in the IVF lab, resulting in a live birth (Fig. 15.1). Cha et al. [3] described the first pregnancy and delivery following IVM of oocytes collected in an unstimulated cycle. Indeed, the technology holds numerous advantages. Fertility medications used for ovarian stimulation are expensive; therefore, an unstimulated cycle means a big cost saving. If the patient is not stimulated, then the risk of OHSS is eliminated, leading to a potential "OHSS-free clinic." Of note, the term "OHSS-free clini-

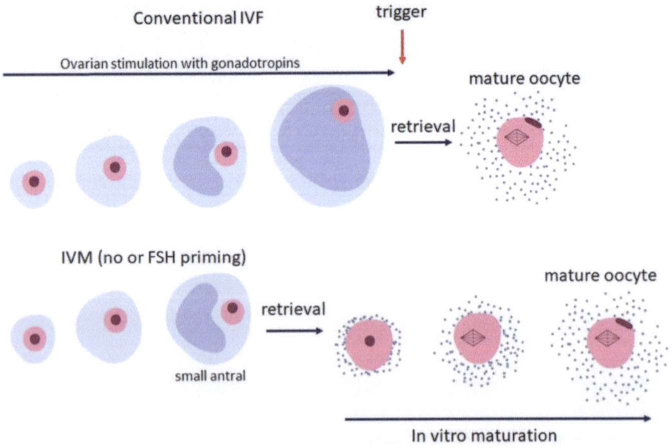

Fig. 15.1 Schematic illustration of an IVM cycle compared with a conventional IVF cycle. (Modified after De Vos et al., J Assist Reprod Genet. 2021;38:1265–1280)

cal environment" was first coined by Kol [4], but in the context of using a GnRH agonist to trigger ovulation, leading to luteolysis. This term was echoed 7 years later by Devroey et al. [5] OHSS is an iatrogenic condition caused by the formation of multiple CL post-ovarian stimulation and ovulation triggering. OHSS can be prevented by quick and irreversible luteolysis, which is almost always the result of GnRH agonist triggering [4]. OHSS can also be prevented by avoiding ovarian stimulation and CL formation, which is the basic premise of IVM. With all these potential advantages, one would expect a swift adoption of the technology; however, this has not been realized yet.

15.3 Clinical Discussion

The IVF lab work associated with IVM is complex, which may be a fair price to pay for a good clinical outcome, but the jury is still out in that respect. For example, Das et al. [6] reported treatment outcomes and rates of OHSS in patients with polycystic ovarian syndrome (PCOS), who underwent assisted conception with either IVM or IVF using GnRH-antagonist protocol. They found a significantly higher live-birth rate in the IVF group compared with the IVM group. As expected, no OHSS was reported in the IVM group.

The IVM technology faces two clinical hurdles: first, the oocyte yield following egg retrieval is lower after IVM compared to conventional IVF ovarian stimulation. In addition, the overall quality of oocytes obtained with IVM culture systems tends to be inferior compared to oocytes retrieved in IVF [7]. The reason for this lies in the technology itself. Immature oocytes retrieved from antral follicles, not exposed to the mid-cycle LH surge, undergo spontaneous meiotic maturation in vitro. This leads to a lack of adequate cytoplasmic maturation, loss of synchronization between nuclear and cytoplasmic maturity, and hence, lower potential for fertilization and lower embryo quality. The proposed clinical solution is to use ovarian stimulation with gonadotropins ("FSH priming") for a few days, followed by triggering ovulation with hCG [8]. This sounds more like "mild ovarian stimulation" than IVM. How many days of FSH stimulation are needed remains a matter of personal decision by different clinicians, which is also pertinent to the use of hCG as a trigger [9]. Since the retrieved follicles are significantly smaller compared with routine IVF, special care is needed to choose the right retrieval needle and aspiration pressure. From the IVF lab perspective, oocyte collection and identification can be a challenge, especially if hCG triggering was not used.

Fresh transfer after IVM is feasible; however, the endometrium is exposed to low estradiol concentrations secreted by the small antral follicles, which is also of short duration. A few days of FSH priming may establish adequate endometrial growth and receptivity. If the endometrium is deemed suboptimal, then a "freeze-all" approach is implemented, followed by a conventional FET protocol.

From the lab work perspective, there is no consensus on the optimal culture media and oocyte maturation protocol to be used in IVM. Monophasic and biphasic methods have been suggested, and different culture medium supplementations were introduced, e.g., serum, FSH, LH/hCG, EGF-like growth factors, and other oocyte-secreted factors. Although IVM has been practiced for many years, research into the optimal combination and concentrations of these supplements in the culture medium still continues.

15.4 IVM in OHSS High-Risk Patients

IVM was suggested as the protocol of choice for women who are at risk of developing OHSS following conventional ovarian stimulation, such as PCOS patients. Indeed, if the ovaries are not stimulated, the hormonal changes that may lead to OHSS are eliminated; therefore, OHSS is prevented. Zheng et al. [10] reported the results of a randomized controlled trial comparing IVM versus standard IVF in women with PCOS. In the IVM group, there were no cases of OHSS, while in the IVF group, ten women (5.7%) had moderate OHSS and one woman (0.6%) had severe OHSS. Vuong et al. [11] performed a randomized controlled trial on 546 patients with high antral follicular count (≥24 follicles in both ovaries), who were obviously at risk for OHSS with conventional ovarian stimulation. In the IVM group, 273 patients underwent one cycle of IVM with a prematuration step. In the IVF group, 273 patients underwent a standard IVF cycle with a GnRH antagonist protocol and GnRH agonist triggering. OHSS did not occur in the IVM group, whereas two cases occurred in the IVF group ("early moderate/severe grade"). Importantly, in both groups, day 3 embryos were vitrified for transfer in a subsequent cycle. Hence, these two OHSS cases underline the possible development of OHSS in spite of using the GnRH agonist trigger and freeze-all strategy. Previous reports confirmed the rare occurrence of OHSS following GnRH agonist trigger, emphasizing that in some patients, quick and irreversible luteolysis is not achieved [12, 13]. However, beyond case reports, high responders may expect only mild symptoms of OHSS after GnRH agonist triggering and freeze-all [14].

GnRH agonist triggering and the "freeze-all" approach have been developed to reduce the risk of OHSS. A systematic review and meta-analysis showed that the pooled incidence of severe OHSS in high-risk women who did not receive any form of luteal phase support was 0% [15]. Hence, most clinicians prefer to use a conventional IVF cycle, with a GnRH antagonist protocol, trigger with a GnRH agonist if OHSS is a concern, and use a "freeze-all" approach rather than the challenging IVM technology. Therefore, the popularity of IVM in OHSS-high-risk patients has declined. What do patients prefer? A partial answer comes from a multicenter discrete choice experiment in the Netherlands, which found that PCOS patients are willing to trade off cancellation rate, number of hormone injections, chance of pregnancy, and costs for a lower risk of OHSS [16]. As mentioned above, FSH priming and hCG trigger in the context of an IVM cycle may expose potential high-responder patients to OHSS, although such an occurrence has not yet been reported.

15.5 Recent Advances

More than 30 years have passed since the successful pregnancy achieved after IVM [3], yet the technology is still not globally practiced. The economic driving force to use IVM is mostly affecting ART centers located mainly in Asia, where patients themselves cover the treatment cost. Therefore, recent scientific literature is rich with reports on improved IVM protocols originating from these countries. Important advances have been described in understanding the impact of different IVM protocols on oocyte developmental outcomes. Improved culture systems have been suggested for cumulus-enclosed immature oocytes that optimally mimic the physiological acquisition of oocyte meiotic competence and cytoplasmic maturity. In this context, an IVM special interest group (IVMSIG) of the American Society for Reproductive Medicine (ASRM) has been established to coordinate research, education, and training in the field of IVM, which may contribute to a better understanding and implementation of the IVM technology in the future.

Recently published studies demonstrate comparable clinical outcomes with IVM or conventional IVF [17]; however, more robust randomized clinical trials are needed to draw firm conclusions in that respect. The novel capacitation in vitro maturation approach (CAPA IVM) seems like an important step in that direction [18]. From the safety point of view, available data suggest that IVM is safe for both patients treated and children born [19].

15.6 Conclusion

IVM is not an experimental technology. IVM has been practiced for decades and is endorsed by professional organizations. In the context of OHSS prevention, IVM is attractive in patients with excessive antral follicle count. In theory, IVM has the potential to replace conventional IVF given its obvious advantages, primarily low cost and improved patient safety. This has not been realized, because the optimal IVM technology has not yet been established. Future research efforts should focus on establishing the optimal patient preparation, oocyte retrieval, and culture system for IVM.

References

1. Edwards R. Maturation in vitro of human ovarian oocytes. Lancet. 1965;286:926–9.
2. Practice Committees of the American Society for Reproductive Medicine, the Society of Reproductive Biologists and Technologists, and the Society for Assisted Reproductive Technology. In vitro maturation: a committee opinion. Fertil Steril. 2021;115:298–304.
3. Cha KY, Koo JJ, Ko JJ, Choi DH, Han SY, Yoon TK. Pregnancy after in vitro fertilization of human follicular oocytes collected from nonstimulated cycles, their culture in vitro and their transfer in a donor oocyte program. Fertil Steril. 1991;55:109–13.
4. Kol S. Luteolysis induced by a gonadotropin-releasing hormone agonist is the key to prevention of ovarian hyperstimulation syndrome. Fertil Steril. 2004;81:1–5.
5. Devroey P, Polyzos NP, Blockeel C. An OHSS-free clinic by segmentation of IVF treatment. Hum Reprod. 2011;26:2593–7.
6. Das M, Son WY, Buckett W, Tulandi T, Holzer H. In-vitro maturation versus IVF with GnRH antagonist for women with polycystic ovary syndrome: treatment outcome and rates of ovarian hyperstimulation syndrome. Reprod Biomed Online. 2014;29:545–51.
7. Gilchrist RB, Smitz J. Oocyte in vitro maturation: physiological basis and application to clinical practice. Fertil Steril. 2023;119:524–39.
8. Son WY, Tan SL. Laboratory and embryological aspects of hCG-primed in vitro maturation cycles for patients with polycystic ovaries. Hum Reprod Update. 2010;16:675–89.
9. Reavey J, Vincent K, Child T, Granne IE. Human chorionic gonadotrophin priming for fertility treatment with in vitro maturation. Cochrane Database Syst Rev. 2016;11:CD008720.
10. Zheng X, Guo W, Zeng L, Zheng D, Yang S, Xu Y, et al. In vitro maturation without gonadotropins versus in vitro fertilization with hyperstimulation in women with polycystic ovary syndrome: a non-inferiority randomized controlled trial. Hum Reprod. 2022;37:242–53.
11. Vuong LN, Ho VNA, Ho TM, Dang VQ, Phung TH, Giang NH, et al. In-vitro maturation of oocytes versus conventional IVF in women with infertility and a high antral follicle count: a randomized non-inferiority controlled trial. Hum Reprod. 2020;35:2537–47.
12. Kol S, Breyzman T. GnRH agonist trigger does not always cause luteolysis: a case report. Reprod Biomed Online. 2016;32(1):132–4.

13. Fatemi HM, Popovic-Todorovic B, Humaidan P, Kol S, Banker M, Devroey P, García-Velasco JA. Severe ovarian hyperstimulation syndrome after gonadotropin-releasing hormone (GnRH) agonist trigger and "freeze-all" approach in GnRH antagonist protocol. Fertil Steril. 2014;101:1008–11.
14. Fernández-Sánchez M, Fatemi H, García-Velasco JA, Heiser PW, Daftary GS, Mannaerts B. Incidence and severity of ovarian hyperstimulation syndrome (OHSS) in high responders after gonadotropin-releasing hormone (GnRH) agonist trigger in "freeze-all" approach. Gynecol Endocrinol. 2023;39:2205952.
15. Ioannidou PG, Bosdou JK, Lainas GT, Lainas TG, Grimbizis GF, Kolibianakis EM. How frequent is severe ovarian hyperstimulation syndrome after GnRH agonist triggering in high-risk women? A systematic review and meta-analysis. Reprod Biomed Online. 2021;42:635–50.
16. Braam SC, de Bruin JP, Mol BWJ, van Wely M. The perspective of women with an increased risk of OHSS regarding the safety and burden of IVF: a discrete choice experiment. Hum Reprod Open. 2020;2020(2):hoz034.
17. Vuong LN, Pham TD, Ho TM, De Vos M. Outcomes of clinical in vitro maturation programs for treating infertility in hyper responders: a systematic review. Fertil Steril. 2023;119:540–9.
18. Vuong LN, Ho VNA, Le AH, Nguyent NT, Pham TD, Nguyen MHN, et al. Hormone-free vs. follicle stimulating hormone-primes infertility treatment of women with polycycstic ovary syndrome using biphasic in vitro maturation: a randomized controlled trial. Fertil Steril. 2025;123:253–261.
19. Strowitzki T, Bruckner T, Roesner S. Maternal and neonatal outcome and children's development after medically assisted reproduction with in-vitro matured oocytes-a systematic review and meta-analysis. Hum Reprod Update. 2021;27:460–73.

Newer Drugs, Interventions and Strategies for an OHSS-Free Practice

16

Jyoti Tripathi and Sulbha Arora

16.1 Introduction

Ovarian hyperstimulation syndrome (OHSS) is a well-known complication of controlled ovarian stimulation (COS). It is difficult to determine the actual incidence of ovarian hyperstimulation due to the lack of a clear definition, although there are several reports that estimate the incidence of moderate-to-severe OHSS to be approximately 1–5% of IVF cycles [1]. Since the advent of assisted reproductive techniques (ART), fertility practitioners and researchers all across the globe have focused on the development of strategies to mitigate the risk of OHSS. Recent advancements in pharmacology, interventions and strategies have been helpful in achieving an OHSS-free practice. There is no fully proven strategy to completely eliminate OHSS; however, there are several modalities which can help reduce the incidence of OHSS. This chapter aims to summarise all the cutting-edge advancements in the field of ART that may help establish an OHSS-free clinic.

J. Tripathi (✉)
Nova IVF Fertility, Indore, Madhya Pradesh, India

S. Arora
Nova IVF Fertility, Mumbai, Maharashtra, India

G. N. Allahbadia et al. (eds.), *Ovarian Hyperstimulation Syndrome (OHSS) Free Clinic*, https://doi.org/10.1007/978-981-95-3289-6_16

16.2 Pharmacological Advancements

Ovarian hyperstimulation can occur in any woman undergoing IVF stimulation. The most important step in the prevention of OHSS is to identify women who are at higher risk of OHSS and to plan individualised treatment protocols.

1. *Stimulation Protocols: GnRH Agonist vs GnRH Antagonist*

Ovarian stimulation protocols during an IVF cycle aim at multifollicular development along with the prevention of premature LH surge. The two most widely used protocols for ovarian stimulation are GnRH agonist and GnRH antagonist protocols. There are multiple studies which have reported that the incidence of OHSS is lower in IVF cycles using an antagonist protocol vs a GnRH agonist protocol, irrespective of the type of trigger used. A Cochrane systematic review and meta-analysis, including 12,212 participants, reported a statistically significant reduction in the incidence of OHSS (odds ratio (OR) 0.61, 95% confidence interval (CI) 0.51–0.72) with the use of GnRH antagonists vs GnRH agonists, although there was no significant difference in live birth and miscarriage rates [2].

2. *Individualised Stimulation Protocols*

Identification of women who are at higher risk of OHSS, based on baseline evaluation and markers of ovarian response, is one of the most crucial steps toward establishing an OHSS-free clinic. This can help in strategizing individualised stimulation protocols, starting with a lower dose of gonadotropin injections in women at risk. An RCT conducted by Simone C Oudshoorn on Individualised vs Standard FSH dosing in women with a predicted hyperresponse in IVF/ICSI reported a lower occurrence of any grade of OHSS with a lower FSH dose (5.2% vs 11.8%, RR 0.44 (95% CI, 0.28–0.71), $P = 0.001$), but the occurrence of severe OHSS did not differ significantly (1.3% vs 1.1%, RR 1.25 (95% CI, 0.38–4.07), $P = 0.728$) [3].

Another systematic review evaluating 20 RCTs which compared individualised gonadotropin dosing on the basis of ovarian reserve testing (ORT) vs standard uniform gonadotropin dosing observed that lower gonadotropin dosing on the basis of ORT decreased the incidence of moderate or severe OHSS (OR 0.58, CI 0.34–1.0), but no significant differences in live birth rates were reported [4].

3. *Utilising Aromatase Inhibitors (AIs) for Ovulation Induction*

AIs like letrozole work by reducing oestrogen production through the inhibition of cytochrome P450 enzymes. This leads to increased pituitary secretion of FSH, which stimulates folliculogenesis. Additionally, the central negative feedback mechanisms remain intact, supporting the theory that it may lower the incidence of OHSS during ovarian stimulation, even though the mechanism for the possible reduction in the risk of OHSS is not completely understood [5]. However, a recent Cochrane review by Franik et al. found no difference in OHSS rates when using AIs compared to other stimulation protocols [6]. As such, their routine use is not recommended.

4. *Gonadotropin-Releasing Hormone (GnRH) Agonist Trigger*

The most important cause of iatrogenic OHSS is the use of hCG for ovarian trigger to induce final oocyte maturation during an IVF cycle. It has been used for this purpose for decades. Due to its long half-life and sustained LH-like activity, it stimulates VEGF from granulosa cells, making it an important prerequisite for OHSS predisposition, even in normoresponder patients.

The advent of a GnRH agonist to induce endogenous LH surge for final oocyte maturation has been a major breakthrough in the field of ART. Substitution of hCG with a GnRH agonist eliminates the risk of OHSS due to its shorter half-life. The LH surge induced by the GnRH agonist lasts for only 24 hours. Over the past decade, GnRH agonists used during the final oocyte maturation have effectively reduced OHSS. A Cochrane review of 17

RCTs with 1847 participants compared GnRH agonists to hCG as the follicular maturation trigger. GnRH agonists significantly reduced OHSS risk (OR 0.15, 95% CI 0.05 to 0.47, n = 989; $I^2 = 42\%$, moderate-quality evidence) but lowered live birth rates (OR 0.47, 95% CI 0.31 to 0.70, n = 532; $I^2 = 56\%$, moderate-quality evidence) and increased early miscarriage rates in fresh autologous cycles. This approach often necessitates a freeze-all strategy [7].

There are reports on the use of a small dose of hCG to overcome the luteal-phase insufficiency, but this also increases the risk of OHSS [8]. Furthermore, frozen embryo transfer cycles have a higher risk of maternal and foetal complications like pre-eclampsia, post-partum haemorrhage and large for gestational age babies [9].

5. *Kisspeptin Agonist Trigger*

Kisspeptin is a naturally occurring peptide that acts on the GnRH neurons which stimulate the hypothalamus to release GnRH, which in turn enhances the secretion of both LH and FSH from the pituitary [10]. It acts as a mediator to integrate feedback from circulating sex steroids to regulate GnRH secretion [11].

The duration of the LH rise induced by a kisspeptin receptor agonist closely resembles that of the endogenous LH surge [12]. However, robust data on its use in IVF treatment are still lacking. Beyond its primary action to stimulate hypothalamic GnRH release, it could potentially have a direct action on the ovary to enhance oocyte maturation [13, 14] and to decrease VEGF secretion and OHSS [15].

A retrospective single centre study compared rates of OHSS following hCG (n = 40), GnRHa (n = 99) or kisspeptin (n = 122) in women at high risk of OHSS (defined as AFC or total number of follicles on day of trigger >23). The odds ratio for developing OHSS was significantly higher following hCG (OR 33.6, 95% CI 12.6–89.5) as well as GnRHa (OR 3.6, 95% CI 1.8–7.1) compared to kisspeptin [16].

6. *Modified hCG Protocols*

Altering the dosage of hCG for triggering final oocyte maturation has been studied by various investigators. An RCT of 80 PCOS patients comparing different doses of urinary hCG in doses of 2500 IU, 5000 IU and 10,000 IU found no significant difference in OHSS rates [17].

In a study by Lin et al. on 164 IVF/ICSI patients comparing urinary hCG in doses of 4000 IU vs 6000 IU, the results found no statistically significant difference in OHSS rates (3.6% vs 4.9%), although significantly lower pregnancy rates were observed in the group that received 4000 IU compared to the one that received 6000 IU (36.5% vs 57.0%) [18].

7. *Recombinant LH for Trigger*

Use of recombinant LH (recLH) to mimic endogenous LH surge for ovulation trigger in high-risk patients is another proposed prevention strategy. recLH has a half-life of 10 hours and also leads to a shorter and/or lower LH peak; thus, it can be helpful in reducing the risk of OHSS. A Cochrane review by Youssef et al. comparing the risk for severe OHSS between recLH and urinary hCG, however, did not show any difference [19].

8. *Dopamine Agonists*

Vascular endothelial growth factor is the key mediator in the pathophysiology of OHSS. It increases vascular permeability. Dopamine agonists have been introduced as a secondary prevention agent in women who have an exaggerated response to COS. Cabergoline is a dopamine agonist which has antiangiogenic properties and prevents the excessive increase in VEGF-mediated vascular permeability encountered with OHSS [20]. Leitao et al. in a systemic review of 7 RCTs reported the efficacy of cabergoline in preventing the occurrence of moderate and severe OHSS (RR 0.38; 95% CI 0.29–0.51) without a negative impact on clinical pregnancy or oocytes retrieved [21].

In the Cochrane review on the effectiveness of cabergoline in the reduction of OHSS by Tang et al., 2 RCTs were included, with 230 women. They found a significant reduction in the incidence of moderate OHSS (OR 0.38; 95% CI 0.19–0.78) with no significant effect on the clinical pregnancy rate and miscarriage rates [22].

Another Cochrane review on the use of dopamine agonists such as cabergoline, quinagolide and bromocriptine, in the context of OHSS, concluded that dopamine agonists probably lowered the risk of moderate or severe OHSS compared to placebo or no intervention in long agonist protocols (OR 0.32, 95% CI 0.23–0.44; 10 studies, 1202 participants; moderate-quality evidence). There was no evidence of an effect of dopamine agonists on live birth rates (OR 0.96, 95% CI 0.60–1.55; 3 studies, 362 participants; low-quality evidence) [23].

Considering the low cost, easy availability, safety and efficacy of dopamine agonists, it is recommended to use them starting either on the day of trigger or day of oocyte collection, as a daily dose of 0.5 mg of cabergoline for 7 or 8 days [24].

9. *Luteal-Phase GnRH Antagonist*

Administration of GnRH antagonist after oocyte retrieval combined with an all-freeze cycle is found to be effective in reducing the progression to OHSS. The luteolytic effect of GnRH antagonist leads to regression of the corpus luteum, suppression of ovarian activity, reduction in ovarian dimensions and thus regression of OHSS.

A prospective study on GnRH antagonist administration for 3 days after oocyte retrieval in a total of 105 patients at a high risk of OHSS found it effective in decreasing the incidence of moderate-to-severe OHSS and faster symptomatic improvement of OHSS (11/61 (18.03%) vs 13/35 (37.14%), $p = 0.03$) [25].

16.3 Freeze-All Strategy

Cryopreservation of all embryos and deferring fresh embryo transfer during the IVF cycle in women at risk of OHSS is helpful in decreasing the incidence of OHSS. Embryo cryopreservation allows avoiding pregnancy and mitigates the risk of late onset OHSS due to the endogenous production of hCG. Several studies have established that the GnRH antagonist protocol combined with GnRH agonist trigger and freeze-all strategy during IVF cycles is a highly effective tool in the prevention of OHSS [26–28].

16.4 Rat Model Studies: Future Avenues in OHSS Prevention

1. *Vasopressin-Induced VEGF Secretion Blockade*

Relcovaptan, a V1A receptor antagonist, is being investigated in rat models as a potential strategy for OHSS prevention by inhibiting vasopressin-induced VEGF secretion. It has been observed that it can inhibit VEGF by modulating vasoconstriction and smooth muscle proliferation. This novel therapy, in the hyperstimulated rat model, has been shown to reduce the concentrations of VEGF-A in the peritoneal fluid, reduce ovarian weight gain and significantly decrease the number of corpora lutea in contrast to control groups. Further research may have promising outcomes in the management protocols for OHSS in the near future [29].

2. *Nintedanib*

Nintedanib is a clinically approved medication for the treatment of non-small cell lung cancer, pulmonary fibrosis and systemic sclerosis-associated interstitial lung disease [30]. It is a tyrosine kinase inhibitor which inhibits multiple receptor tyrosine kinases (RTKs) like vascular endothelial growth factor receptors (VEGFRs), fibroblast growth factor receptors (FGFRs) and platelet-derived growth factor receptors (PDGFRs). These three receptors play a very crucial role in promoting angiogenesis [31]. Hence, this drug has gained interest and is being studied in mouse models as a treatment option for managing OHSS.

A study by Shutian Jiang found that when Nintedanib was given after hCG trigger, it significantly alleviated the symptoms of OHSS in the mouse model (weight change, $P < 0.0001$; ovarian weight, $P < 0.0001$, peritoneal exudation level, $P < 0.01$). It was also observed that it inhibited the proliferation of the corpus luteum (number, $P < 0.001$; diameter, $P < 0.0001$) and luteal vessel ($P < 0.0001$) development [32]. The study concluded that owing to its strong angiogenesis inhibition, it reduces the vascular permeability induced by VEGF to alleviate the severity of OHSS symptoms. Since it inhibits the corpus luteal development and has a luteolytic effect, a fresh embryo transfer is not ideal when it is used, and a freeze-all cycle is recommended.

The initial results are promising, but more studies are still needed to establish its efficacy and safety for clinical use.

3. *Aflibercept*

Aflibercept is an antiangiogenic medication. It is a fusion protein which is produced using recombinant DNA technology [33]. It acts as a decoy receptor, preventing the binding of VEGF to its natural receptor and thereby inhibiting angiogenesis. It is approved for the treatment of maculopathy and metastatic colorectal cancer. Considering the angiogenic pathophysiology of OHSS, this drug has gained attention as a possible treatment for OHSS.

An experimental study conducted in the rat model comparing aflibercept and cabergoline in the prevention and treatment of ovarian hyperstimulation found that aflibercept is more efficacious in reducing vascular permeability and VEGF expression in OHSS than cabergoline [34]. Further clinical trials are needed to establish its use in the treatment of OHSS.

16.5 Conclusion

Ovarian hyperstimulation is a potentially preventable yet one of the most challenging complications associated with assisted reproductive technology (ART). Since the advent of ART over the decades, the paradigm has shifted from managing OHSS to the prevention of OHSS. The combination of clinical assessment of at-risk women, use of individualised stimulation protocols, strategic use of modern pharmacological and non-pharmacological interventions like GnRH antagonist protocols, GnRH agonist trigger and freeze-all strategies has significantly reduced the incidence of OHSS. Novel agents such as kisspeptin triggers, along with emerging therapies like angiogenesis inhibitors, show promise for future application. Further research and clinical trials are essential to establish evidence-based protocols and achieve an OHSS-free practice.

References

1. Steward RG, Lan L, Shah AA, Yeh JS, Price TM, Goldfarb JM, et al. Oocyte number as a predictor for ovarian hyperstimulation syndrome and live birth: an analysis of 256,381 in vitro fertilization cycles. Fertil Steril. 2014;101:967–73.
2. Al-Inany HG, Youssef MA, Ayeleke RO, Brown J, Lam WS, Broekmans FJ. Gonadotrophin-releasing hormone antagonists for assisted reproductive technology. Cochrane Database Syst Rev. 2016;4:CD001750.
3. Oudshoorn SC, van Tilborg TC, Eijkemans MJC, Oosterhuis GJE, Friederich J, van Hooff MHA, et al. Individualized versus standard FSH dosing in women starting IVF/ICSI: an RCT. Part 2: the predicted hyper responder. Hum Reprod. 2017;32:2506–14.
4. Lensen SF, Wilkinson J, Leijdekkers JA, La Marca A, Mol BWJ, Marjoribanks J, et al. Individualised gonadotropin dose selection using markers of ovarian reserve for women undergoing in vitro fertilisation plus intracytoplasmic sperm injection (IVF/ICSI). Cochrane Database Syst Rev. 2018;2:CD012693.
5. Lee VCY, Ledger W. Aromatase inhibitors for ovulation induction and ovarian stimulation. Clin Endocrinol. 2011;74(5):537–46.
6. Franik S, Kremer JA, Nelen WL, Farquhar C. Aromatase inhibitors for subfertile women with polycystic ovary syndrome. Cochrane Database Systematic Rev. 2014;2:CD010287.
7. Youssef MA, Van der Veen F, Al-Inany HG, Mochtar MH, Griesinger G, Nagi Mohesen M, Aboulfoutouh I, van Wely M. Gonadotropin-releasing hormone agonist versus HCG for oocyte triggering in antagonist-assisted reproductive technology. The. Cochrane Database Syst Rev. 2014;10:CD008046.
8. Abbara A, Clarke SA, Dhillo WS. Novel concepts for inducing final oocyte maturation in in vitro fertilization treatment. Endocrine Rev. 2018;39:593–628.
9. Sha T, Yin X, Cheng W, Massey IY. Pregnancy-related complications and perinatal outcomes resulting from transfer of cryopreserved versus fresh

embryos in vitro fertilization: a meta-analysis. Fertility Sterility. 2018;109:330–42.
10. Clarke H, Dhillo WS, Jayasena CN. Comprehensive review on kisspeptin and its role in reproductive disorders. Endocrinol Metab. 2015;30:124.
11. Abbara A, Clarke SA, Dhillo WS. Clinical potential of kisspeptin in reproductive health. Trends Mol Med. 2021;27:807–23.
12. Abbara A, Eng PC, Phylactou M, Clarke SA, Richardson R, Sykes CM, et al. Kisspeptin receptor agonist has therapeutic potential for female reproductive disorders. J Clin Invest. 2020;130:6739–53.
13. Ruohonen ST, Gaytan F, Usseglio Gaudi A, Velasco I, Kukoricza K, Perdices-Lopez C, et al. Selective loss of kisspeptin signaling in oocytes causes progressive premature ovulatory failure. Hum Reprod. 2022;37:806–21.
14. Owens LA, Abbara A, Lerner A, O'Floinn S, Christopoulos G, Khanjani S, et al. The direct and indirect effects of kisspeptin-54 on granulosa lutein cell function. Hum Reprod. 2018;33:292–302.
15. Abbara A, Hunjan T, Ho VNA, Clarke SA, Comninos AN, Izzi-Engbeaya C, et al. Endocrine requirements for oocyte maturation following hCG, GnRH agonist, and kisspeptin during IVF treatment. Front Endocrinol. 2020;11:537205.
16. Abbara A, Islam R, Clarke SA, Jeffers L, Christopoulos G, Comninos AN, et al. Clinical parameters of ovarian hyperstimulation syndrome following different hormonal triggers of oocyte maturation in IVF treatment. Clin Endocrinol. 2018;88:920–7.
17. Kolibianakis EM, Papanikolaou EG, Tournaye H, Camus M, Van Steirteghem AC, Devroey P. Triggering final oocyte maturation using different doses of human chorionic gonadotropin: a randomized pilot study in patients with polycystic ovary syndrome treated with gonadotropin-releasing hormone antagonists and recombinant follicle-stimulating hormone. Fertil Steril. 2007;88(5):1382–8.
18. Lin H, Wang W, Li Y, Chen X, Yang D, Zhang Q. Triggering final oocyte maturation with reduced doses of hCG in IVF/ICSI: a prospective, randomized and controlled study. Eur J Obstet Gynecol Reprod Biol. 2011;159(1):143–7.
19. Youssef MA, Al-Inany HG, Aboulghar M, Mansour R, Abou-Setta AM. Recombinant versus urinary human chorionic gonadotrophin for final oocyte maturation triggering in IVF and ICSI cycles. Cochrane Database Syst Rev. 2011:4 CD003719.
20. Garcia-Velasco JA. How to avoid ovarian hyperstimulation syndrome: a new indication for dopamine agonists. Reprod Biomed Online. 2009;18(2):S71–5.
21. Leitao V, Moroni RM, Seko L, Nastri CO, Martins WP. Cabergoline for the prevention of ovarian hyperstimulation syndrome: systematic review and meta-analysis of randomized controlled trials. Fertil Steril. 2014;101(3):664–75.

22. Tang H, Hunter T, Hu Y, Zhai SD, Sheng X, Hart RJ. Cabergoline for preventing ovarian hyperstimulation syndrome. Cochrane Database Syst Rev. 2012;2. CD008605
23. Tang H, Mourad SM, Wang A, Zhai SD, Hart RJ. Dopamine agonists for preventing ovarian hyperstimulation syndrome. The. Cochrane Database Syst Rev. 2021;4(4):CD008605.
24. Kasum M, Vrčić H, Stanić P, et al. Dopamine agonists in prevention of ovarian hyperstimulation syndrome. Gynecol Endocrinol. 2014;30(12):845–9.
25. Zeng C, Shang J, Jin AM, Wu PL, Li X, Xue Q. The effect of luteal GnRH antagonist on moderate and severe early ovarian hyperstimulation syndrome during in vitro fertilization treatment: a prospective cohort study. Arch Gynecol Obstet. 2019;300:223–33.
26. D'Angelo A. Ovarian hyperstimulation syndrome prevention strategies: cryopreservation of all embryos. Semin Reprod Med. 2010;28:513–8.
27. D'Angelo A, Amso N. Embryo freezing for preventing ovarian hyperstimulation syndrome. Cochrane Database Syst Rev. 2007:CD002806.
28. Devroey P, Adriaensen P. OHSS free clinic. Facts Views Vis Obgyn. 2011;3:43–5.
29. Cenksoy C, Cenksoy PO, Erdem O, Sancak B, Gursoy R. A potential novel strategy, inhibition of vasopressin-induced VEGF secretion by relcovaptan, for decreasing the incidence of ovarian hyperstimulation syndrome in the hyperstimulated rat model. European J Obs Gynecol Reprod Biol. 2014;174(1):86–90.
30. Wollin L, Distler JHW, Redente EF, et al. Potential of nintedanib in treatment of progressive fibrosing interstitial lung diseases. Eur Respir J. 2019;54(3):1900161.
31. Lamb YN. Nintedanib: a review in fibrotic interstitial lung diseases. Drugs. 2021;81(5):575–86.
32. Jiang S, Li W, Zhao X, Chen L, Kuang Y. Nintedanib treatment after ovulation is an effective therapeutic strategy for the alleviation of ovarian Hyperstimulation syndrome (OHSS) in a mouse model. Drug Des Devel Ther. 2022;18(16):397–411.
33. Chung C, Pherwani N. Ziv-aflibercept: a novel angiogenesis inhibitor for the treatment of metastatic colorectal cancer. Am J Health Syst Pharm. 2013;70:1887–96.
34. Çağlayan A, Berna D, Seval YE, Fuad A. Aflibercept suppresses ovarian hyperstimulation syndrome: an experimental study in rats. Rev Assoc Med Bras (1992) 2023;69(11):e20230789.

Freeze-All for All Is the Way Ahead

17

Murat Berkkanoglu, Kevin Coetzee, and Kemal Ozgur

17.1 Introduction

Ovarian hyperstimulation syndrome (OHSS) is a significant adverse outcome of assisted reproduction technology (ART) treatments utilizing ovarian stimulation, with enlarged ovaries and acute fluid shift from the intravascular to the interstitial space or third space being characteristic of this condition. These primary symptoms are associated with bloating, ascites, pleural effusion, hemoconcentration, hypercoagulability, electrolytic imbalance, venous thromboembolism, and decreased organ perfusion.

In 1989, OHSS was first classified as a mild, moderate, or severe condition [1]. Thereafter, the classification has been modified by including ultrasonographic measurements of the stimulated ovaries [2]. In a 2006 study, it was reported that most cases presented as mild forms, with only 3–8% transforming into moderate or severe OHSS in in vitro fertilization (IVF) cycles [3].

M. Berkkanoglu
Antalya IVF Centre, Antalya, Turkey

Department of Obstetrics and Gynecology, Istanbul Atlas University, School of Medicine, Istanbul, Turkey

K. Coetzee · K. Ozgur (✉)
Antalya IVF Centre, Antalya, Turkey

G. N. Allahbadia et al. (eds.), *Ovarian Hyperstimulation Syndrome (OHSS) Free Clinic*, https://doi.org/10.1007/978-981-95-3289-6_17

In 2017, the European Society of Human Reproduction and Embryology (ESHRE), in their report on ART procedures in Europe, reported on cycles performed in 39 participating countries, indicating that the incidence rate for OHSS in all reported cycles was 0.2% [4]. This large difference in incidence rates could be due to underestimation/underreporting or variability in the classification of OHSS by physicians. Moreover, it could also be due to the many preventative strategies that have recently been introduced in clinical practice worldwide, with these possibly reducing the incidence of this potentially life-threatening condition. OHSS often occurs due to an excessive response to ovarian stimulation, although it can sometimes be an idiosyncratic reaction to gonadotropins, with spontaneous OHSS incidents not related to ovarian stimulation also reported [5, 6]. Moreover, young women with low body mass indices and polycystic ovaries may have an increased OHSS risk [7].

The exact underlying molecular pathophysiology of OHSS is not fully understood; however, several distinct molecular pathways have been identified for research. Firstly, human chorionic gonadotropin (hCG) has greater biological affinity than luteinizing hormone (LH) for the LH receptor and a longer half-life activity, with hCG activating numerous downstream events [8]. Secondly, there is an increased expression of vascular endothelial growth factor (VEGF), with VEGF hyperactivation associated with a massive increase in vascular permeability [9]. Other molecular pathways also activated include the angiotensin–renin system, the kallikrein–kinin system, the release of transforming growth factor, histamine, prolactin, prostaglandins, and insulin-like growth factors [10–16].

17.2 Interventions

In recent decades, various strategies have been implemented in clinical practice to prevent this potentially life-threatening condition. In a recent systematic review of preventative interventions to reduce the incidence and severity of OHSS, approximately 40 different interventions were examined, [17] including treatment alternatives such as mild ovarian stimulation, natural ovarian stimulation, progestin-primed ovarian stimulation, GnRH-ant ovarian stimulation, alternative follicle stimulation drugs, step-down FSH stimulation, alternative trigger types and doses, cycle cancellation, cycle coasting, elective cryopreservation, elective single embryo transfer, in vitro maturation of oocytes, intensified luteal-phase support, luteal-phase support with hCG, luteal-phase support with GnRH-a, and luteal-phase support with progesterone, pretreatments such as ovarian drilling, metformin, oral contraceptives, insulin sensitizing drugs, melatonin, and vitamin D, add-ons such as aspirin, LH, letrozole, OHSS mediators such as calcium infusion, cabergoline, diosmin, dopaminergic agonists, glucocorticoid, inositol, ketoconazole, volume expanders with albumin, and volume expanders with hydroxyethyl starch and personalization of preventative interventions including preventative monitoring and surveillance, and predictive models. [17] Only the interventions applied in randomized controlled trials were assessed by the systematic review and meta-analysis [17].

In the past, cancellation of the stimulation cycle was the intervention most often used to prevent OHSS, with cancellation continuing to be an intervention option, especially when elective cryopreservation of embryos is not possible [18]. Aspirin is commonly used as a supplemental prophylactic medication because it can inhibit the activity of the cyclooxygenase-1 enzyme, decrease platelet activity, and reduce the risk of blood clotting. However, a recent double-blind placebo-controlled RCT reported that there was no difference in the incidence of moderate-to-severe OHSS between the low-dose aspirin and placebo groups of PCOS patients [19]. Inositol, because of its involvement in numerous molecular signaling processes, has also been investigated; [20] however, in a recent double-blind RCT of PCOS patients, no significant difference in OHSS incidence was found between the myo-inositol and metformin pretreatment groups [21].

A randomized controlled study investigating volume expansion using human albumin found that human albumin did not prevent or reduce the risk of severe OHSS [22]. In a Cochrane systematic review, it was reported that dopamine agonists might reduce the incidence of moderate or severe OHSS compared to placebo. Moreover, there is still uncertainty regarding associated adverse events and pregnancy outcomes, including reduced live birth and clinical pregnancy, and increased miscarriage [7]. Metformin, with its insulin-sensitized anti-inflammatory and anti-androgenic effects [23], is a commonly used medication in the prevention of OHSS and the reduction of OHSS severity. In a meta-analysis of studies investigating the use of metformin supplementation in GnRH-a IVF cycles, it was reported that metformin supplementation significantly reduced OHSS risk [24]. Moreover, this reduction of OHSS risk could not be replicated in GnRH-ant IVF cycles [24]. Unfortunately, many of the other medications proposed and introduced into clinical practice have resulted in the reporting of inconsistent abilities to prevent or reduce OHSS.

Some additional alternative strategies using modified stimulation protocols have been proposed to prevent OHSS. In the coasting strategy (1), gonadotropin administration is suspended, and the hCG trigger is delayed until serum estradiol levels have reduced significantly [25]. A meta-analysis demonstrated that coasting effectively reduced OHSS risk [26]. However, there was insufficient evidence to assess the procedure's efficacy in terms of live birth [26]. In the step-down FSH dose strategy (2), the daily dose of FSH is decreased in a step-down manner to optimize safety and cycle outcomes during ovarian stimulation. In a systematic review, it was concluded that decreasing the r-FSH dose during the mid-follicular phase of the ovarian stimulation may reduce the occurrence of OHSS as compared to a fixed FSH dose [27]. In the mild ovarian stimulation strategy (3), the ovaries are stimulated with lower doses of gonadotropins than those used in conventional ovarian stimulations. In a recent meta-analysis, patients receiving mild stimulation were found to have a lower OHSS risk, which was defined as the administration of daily gonadotropin doses of ≤150 IU as compared to normal and hyper-responder controls receiving a higher conventional stimulation gonadotropin doses (>150 UI) [28]. However, this strategy did not lower the OHSS risk in poor responders [28]. Furthermore no difference was detected among normal, poor, and hyper-responders in terms of live birth rates [28]. However, in poor and normal responders undergoing mild stimulation as compared to conventional ovarian stimulation, a reduction in the number of oocytes retrieved was reported. In the hCG trigger dose strategy (4), the dose of the hCG trigger was decreased to reduce OHSS risk [29]. In a GnRH-a administration strategy (5), GnRH-a triggers were used for final oocyte maturation in ovarian stimulation cycles downregulated with a GnRH-ant. A recent systematic review with meta-analysis showed that the GnRH-a trigger has a lower risk for the OHSS compared to an hCG trigger for final oocyte maturation [30]; however, there was a reduction in live birth and ongoing pregnancy rates and an increase in early miscarriage rates in fresh autologous transfer cycles after GnRH-a triggering [30]. The freeze-all strategy (6), which is the elective freezing of all embryos obtained in an IVF cycle, has become the current cornerstone strategy for the prevention of OHSS. A recent meta-analysis indicated that OHSS was significantly reduced in elective frozen embryo transfer cycles compared to routine fresh ET cycles [31–33]. In addition, there has been a significant increase in freeze-all cycles because the cumulative rate of live births increases with an increasing number of oocytes retrieved [34].

Consequently, the freeze-all strategy seems to be replacing all other previously investigated interventions, as well as the previously regarded cornerstone strategy, in which drug doses were personalized. However, the freeze-all strategy does not eliminate OHSS, even when final oocyte maturation is triggered with GnRH-a [35, 36]. Moreover, all IVF clinics are not equally skilled in performing embryo vitrification and warming procedures; patients may be dissatisfied with a longer time to pregnancy, and FET may be associated with increased preeclampsia risks [31].

Therefore, if fresh ET is the transfer strategy of choice, then the best approach for decreasing OHSS risk might be to tailor the starting gonadotropin dose according to patient-specific mathematical algorithms. In this approach, the preferred goal of controlled ovarian stimulation would be to obtain an optimal rather than a maximal number of oocytes, and to achieve a similar live birth rate rather than a similar cumulative live birth rate. The mathematical algorithms are usually based on antral follicle count, ovarian volume, ovarian stromal blood flow detected by Doppler ultrasound (total Doppler score), age, smoking habits, body weight, body mass index, basal FSH level, and AMH [37–41]. A recent systematic review and network meta-analysis indicated that mathematical algorithm-based individualization of gonadotropin starting dose and the freeze-all strategy in normal responders similarly reduced OHSS when compared with conventional treatments [42]. In addition, a recent Cochrane database systematic review suggested that the starting-dose algorithms reduced the incidence of moderate or severe OHSS when compared to a standard starting dose of 150 IU and also resulted in fewer cancellations for hyperresponse [43].

17.3 Conclusion

OHSS is an iatrogenic complication of ovarian stimulations triggered by either exogenous or endogenous hCG in assisted reproductive technology treatments, with severe forms being life-threatening, leading to hemoconcentration, thromboembolic risk, ascites formation, pleural effusion, and an increased risk of ovarian torsion [36].

The treatment approach chosen should balance the desire for pregnancy with the desire to protect patient safety, with treatment approaches upholding the desire for having an OHSS-free clinic in the future. While the use of GnRH-a triggers and freeze-all IVF treatments could be the ultimate OHSS risk reduction strategy, the combined strategy might not eliminate OHSS [35, 36]. Although recent evidence suggests that there is an increased risk of preeclampsia if a pregnancy is achieved in a frozen embryo transfer cycle, especially in hormonal replacement therapy cycles without corpus lutea, the evidence also suggests that the incidence of the complication could possibly be lowered by transferring frozen embryos in true natural cycles, modified natural cycles, or stimulated cycles with existing corpus lutea [44].

On the other hand, if there is still a desire for fresh embryo transfer, tailoring the starting gonadotropin dose according to patient-specific mathematical algorithms could help lower OHSS risk. In this approach, an optimal oocyte number rather than a maximal oocyte number is the preferred outcome, which would achieve a similar live birth rate compared with the freeze-all strategy. Moreover, since cumulative live birth is the desired pregnancy outcome, which increases with increasing number of oocytes retrieved, freeze-all IVF with frozen embryo transfer would be the most effective treatment approach [34].

References

1. Golan A, Ron-el R, Herman A, SoKer Y, Weinraub Z, Caspi E. Ovarian hyperstimulation syndrome: an update review. Obstet Gynecol Surv. 1989;44(6):430–40.
2. Rabau E, David A, Serr DM, Mashiach S, Lunenfeld B. Human menopausal gonadotropins for anovulation and sterility. Results of 7 years of treatment. Am J Obstet Gynecol. 1967;98(1):92–8.
3. Royal College of Obstetricians and Gynaecologists (RCOG). The management of ovarian hyperstimulation syndrome. London (UK): Royal College of Obstetricians and Gynaecologists (RCOG). Green-top Guideline No 5 2006.
4. European IVF-Monitoring Consortium (EIM) for the European Society of Human Reproduction and Embryology (ESHRE), Wyns C, De Geyter C, Calhaz-Jorge C, Kupka MS, Motrenko T, Smeenk J, Bergh C, Tandler-Schneider A, Rugescu IA, Vidakovic S, Goossens V. ART in Europe, 2017: results generated from European registries by ESHRE. Hum Reprod Open. 2021;3:hoab026.
5. Humaidan P, Nelson SM, Devroey P, Coddington CC, Schwartz LB, Gordon K, Frattarelli JL, Tarlatzis BC, Fatemi HM, Lutjen P, et al. Ovarian hyperstimulation syndrome: review and new classification criteria for reporting in clinical trials. Hum Reprod. 2016;31:1997–2004.
6. Dey AK, Dubey A, Mittal K, Kale S. Spontaneous ovarian hyperstimulation syndrome—understanding the dilemma. Gynecol Endocrinol. 2015;31:587–9.
7. Tang H, Mourad SM, Wang A, Zhai SD, Hart RJ. Dopamine agonists for preventing ovarian hyperstimulation syndrome. Cochrane Database Syst Rev. 2021;4(4):CD008605. https://doi.org/10.1002/14651858.CD008605.pub4.
8. Nastri CO, Ferriani RA, Rocha IA, Martins WP. Ovarian hyperstimulation syndrome: pathophysiology and prevention. J Assist Reprod Genet. 2010;27:121–8.
9. Miller I, Chuderland D, Grossman H, Ron-El R, Ben-Ami I, Shalgi R. The dual role of PEDF in the pathogenesis of OHSS: negating both

angiogenic and inflammatory pathways. J Clin Endocrinol Metab. 2016;101:4699–709.
10. Manno M, Tomei F. Renin-angiotensin system activation during severe OHSS: cause or effect? Fertil Steril. 2008;89:488.
11. Kobayashi H, Okada Y, Asahina T, Gotoh J, Terao T. The kallikrein-kinin system, but not vascular endothelial growth factor, plays a role in the increased vascular permeability associated with ovarian hyperstimulation syndrome. J Mol Endocrinol. 1998;20:363–74.
12. Dang X, Fang L, Jia Q, Wu Z, Guo Y, Liu B, Cheng JC, Sun YP. TGF-_1 upregulates secreted protein acidic and rich in cysteine expression in human granulosa-lutein cells: a potential mechanism for the pathogenesis of ovarian hyperstimulation syndrome. Cell Commun Signal. 2023;21:101.
13. Nastri CO, Teixeira DM, Moroni RM, Leitão VM, Martins WP. Ovarian hyperstimulation syndrome: pathophysiology, staging, prediction and prevention. Ultrasound Obstet Gynecol. 2015;45:377–93.
14. Kwik M, Maxwell E. Pathophysiology, treatment and prevention of ovarian hyperstimulation syndrome. Curr Opin Obstet Gynecol. 2016;28:236–41.
15. Gómez R, Soares SR, Busso C, Garcia-Velasco JA, Simón C, Pellicer A. Physiology and pathology of ovarian hyperstimulation syndrome. Semin Reprod Med. 2010;28:448–57.
16. Palumbo A, Ávila J, Naftolin F. The ovarian renin-angiotensin system (OVRAS): a major factor in ovarian function and disease. Reprod Sci. 2016;23:1644–55.
17. Palomba S, Costanzi F, Nelson SM, Besharat A, Caserta D, Humaidan P. Beyond the umbrella: a systematic review of the interventions for the prevention of and reduction in the incidence and severity of Ovarian Hyperstimulation syndrome in patients who undergo in vitro fertilization treatments. Int J Mol Sci. 2023;24(18):14185.
18. Bosch E, Broer S, Griesinger G, Grynberg M, Humaidan P, Kolibianakis E, Kunicki M, La Marca A, Lainas G, et al. ESHRE guideline: Ovarian stimulation for IVF/ICSI. Hum Reprod Open. 2020;2020:hoaa009.
19. Namavar Jahromi B, Zolghadri J, Rahmani E, Alipour S, Anvar Z, Zarei A, Keramati P. Effect of low-dose aspirin on the development of ovarian hyperstimulation syndrome and outcomes of assisted reproductive techniques in the women with PCOS, a randomized double-blinded clinical trial. Taiwan J Obstet Gynecol. 2019;58:255–60.
20. Berridge MJ. The inositol trisphosphate/calcium signaling pathway in health and disease. Physiol Rev. 2016;96:1261–96.
21. Rajasekaran K, Malhotra N, Mahey R, Khadgawat R, Kalaivani M. Myoinositol versus metformin pretreatment in GnRH antagonist cycle for women with PCOS undergoing IVF: a double-blinded randomized controlled study. Gynecol Endocrinol. 2022;38:140–7.

22. Isikoglu M, Berkkanoglu M, Senturk Z, Ozgur K. Human albumin does not prevent ovarian hyperstimulation syndrome in assisted reproductive technology program: a prospective randomized placebo-controlled double blind study. Fertil Steril. 2007;88(4):982–5.
23. Palomba S, Falbo A, Zullo F, Orio F Jr. Evidence-based and potential benefits of metformin in the polycystic ovary syndrome: a comprehensive review. Endocr Rev. 2009;30:1–50.
24. Tso LO, Costello MF, Albuquerque LET, Andriolo RB, Macedo CR. Metformin treatment before and during IVF or ICSI in women with polycystic ovary syndrome. Cochrane Database Syst Rev. 2020;12:CD006105.
25. Delvigne A, Rozenberg S. A qualitative systematic review of coasting, a procedure to avoid ovarian hyperstimulation syndrome in IVF patients. Hum Reprod Update. 2002;8:291–6.
26. D'Angelo A, Amso NN, Hassan R. Coasting (withholding gonadotrophins) for preventing ovarian hyperstimulation syndrome. Cochrane Database Syst Rev. 2017;5:CD002811.
27. Fatemi H, Bilger W, Denis D, Griesinger G, La Marca A, Longobardi S, Mahony M, Yin X, D'Hooghe T. Dose adjustment of follicle-stimulating hormone (FSH) during ovarian stimulation as part of medically-assisted reproduction in clinical studies: a systematic review covering 10 years (2007–2017). Reprod Biol Endocrinol. 2021;19:68.
28. Datta AK, Maheshwari A, Felix N, Campbell S, Nargund G. Mild versus conventional ovarian stimulation for IVF in poor, normal and hyperresponders: a systematic review and meta-analysis. Hum Reprod Update. 2021;27:229–53.
29. Ovarian Stimulation TEGGO, Bosch E, Broer S, Griesinger G, Grynberg M, Humaidan P, Kolibianakis E, Kunicki M, La Marca A, Lainas G, et al. ESHRE guideline: Ovarian stimulation for IVF/ICSI. Hum Reprod Open. 2020;2020:hoaa009.
30. Youssef MA, Van der Veen F, Al-Inany HG, Mochtar MH, Griesinger G, Nagi Mohesen M, Aboulfoutouh I, van Wely M. Gonadotropin-releasing hormone agonist versus HCG for oocyte triggering in antagonistassisted reproductive technology. Cochrane Database Syst Rev. 2014;4:CD008046.
31. Roque M, Haahr T, Geber S, Esteves SC, Humaidan P. Fresh versus elective frozen embryo transfer in IVF/ICSI cycles: a systematic review and meta-analysis of reproductive outcomes. Hum Reprod Update. 2019;25:2–14.
32. Bosdou JK, Venetis CA, Tarlatzis BC, Grimbizis GF, Kolibianakis EM. Higher probability of live-birth in high, but not normal, responders after first frozen-embryo transfer in a freeze-only cycle strategy compared to fresh-embryo transfer: a meta-analysis. Hum Reprod. 2019;34:491–505.

33. Zaat T, Zagers M, Mol F, Goddijn M, van Wely M, Mastenbroek S. Fresh versus frozen embryo transfers in assisted reproduction. Cochrane Database Syst Rev. 2021;2:CD011184.
34. Polyzos NP, Drakopoulos P, Parra J, Pellicer A, Santos-Ribeiro S, Tournaye H, Bosch E, Garcia-Velasco J. Cumulative live birth rates according to the number of oocytes retrieved after the first ovarian stimulation for in vitro fertilization/intracytoplasmic sperm injection: a multicenter multinational analysis including approximately 15,000 women. Fertil Steril. 2018;110:661–70.
35. Fatemi HM, Popovic-Todorovic B, Humaidan P, Kol S, Banker M, Devroey P, García-Velasco JA. Severe ovarian hyperstimulation syndrome after gonadotropin-releasing hormone (GnRH) agonist trigger and "freeze-all" approach in GnRH antagonist protocol. Fertil Steril. 2014;101:1008–11.
36. Berkkanoglu M, Coetzee K, Bulut H, Ozgur K. Risk of ovarian torsion is reduced in GnRH agonist triggered freeze-all cycles: a retrospective cohort study. J Obstet Gynaecol. 2019;39(2):212–7.
37. Popovic-Todorovic B, Loft A, Bredkjaeer HE, Bangsbøll S, Nielsen IK, Andersen AN. A prospective randomized clinical trial comparing an individual dose of recombinant FSH based on predictive factors versus a 'standard' dose of 150 IU/day in 'standard' patients undergoing IVF/ICSI treatment. Hum Reprod. 2003;18:2275–82.
38. Nyboe Andersen A, Nelson SM, Fauser BC, García-Velasco JA, Klein BM, Arce JC. ESTHER-1 study group. Individualized versus conventional ovarian stimulation for in vitro fertilization: a multicenter, randomized, controlled, assessor-blinded, phase 3 noninferiority trial. Fertil Steril. 2017;107:387–96.
39. Bosch E, Havelock J, Martin FS, Rasmussen BB, Klein BM, Mannaerts B, Arce JC. ESTHER-2 Study Group. Follitropin delta in repeated ovarian stimulation for IVF: a controlled, assessor-blind phase 3 safety trial. Reprod Biomed Online. 2019;38:195–205.
40. Ishihara O, Arce JC. For the Japanese Follitropin Delta phase 3 trial (STORK) group. Individualized follitropin delta dosing reduces OHSS risk in Japanese IVF/ICSI patients: a randomized controlled trial. Reprod Biomed Online. 2021;42:909–18.
41. Qiao J, Zhang Y, Liang X, Ho T, Huang H-Y, Kim S-K, Goethberg M, Mannaerts B, Arce JC. On behalf of the Asian follitropin delta phase 3 trial (GRAPE) group. A randomised controlled trial to clinically validate follitropin delta in its individualised dosing regimen for ovarian stimulation in Asian IVF/ICSI patients. Hum Reprod. 2021;36:2452–62.
42. Marino A, Gullo S, Sammartano F, Volpes A, Allegra A. Algorithm-based individualization methodology of the starting gonadotropin dose in IVF/ICSI and the freeze-all strategy prevent OHSS equally in normal responders: a systematic review and network meta-analysis of the evidence. J Assist Reprod Genet. 2022;39(7):1583–601.

43. Ngwenya O, Lensen SF, Vail A, Mol BWJ, Broekmans FJ, Wilkinson J. Individualised gonadotropin dose selection using markers of ovarian reserve for women undergoing in vitro fertilisation plus intracytoplasmic sperm injection (IVF/ICSI). Cochrane Database Syst Rev. 2024;1(1):CD012693.
44. Niu Y, Suo L, Zhao D, Wang Y, Miao R, Zou J, Han X, Chen Z, Li Y, Wei D. Is artificial endometrial preparation more associated with early-onset or late-onset preeclampsia after frozen embryo transfer? J Assist Reprod Genet. 2023;40(5):1045–54.

18 Is There an Ideal Stimulation Protocol for an OHSS-Free Clinic?

Gautam Nand Allahbadia,
Akanksha Allahbadia Gupta,
and Swati Gautam Allahbadia

18.1 Introduction and Rationale

Ovarian hyperstimulation syndrome (OHSS) has long cast a shadow over the otherwise remarkable advances in assisted reproduction. Originally considered an unavoidable risk associated with controlled ovarian stimulation, OHSS has been responsible for thousands of emergency hospitalizations, life-threatening complications, and at least a few maternal deaths across the globe. Its unpredictability, potential severity, and ethical implications have led many to question whether such iatrogenic risk is justifiable in elective fertility treatment.

G. N. Allahbadia (✉)
Allahbadia Fertility Clinic, Dubai, United Arab Emirates
e-mail: allahbadia@allahbadiaivf.com

A. A. Gupta
Sumitra Hospital, Noida, Uttar Pradesh, India

S. G. Allahbadia
Rotunda – The Center for Human Reproduction Wadala (West),
Mumbai, Maharashtra, India

G. N. Allahbadia et al. (eds.), *Ovarian Hyperstimulation Syndrome (OHSS) Free Clinic*, https://doi.org/10.1007/978-981-95-3289-6_18

By 2025, the reproductive medicine community has witnessed a paradigm shift. OHSS, once considered a necessary evil of assisted reproductive technology (ART), is now widely acknowledged to be almost entirely preventable with appropriate stimulation strategies and embryo handling protocols. This evolution has been driven by a cascade of innovations: the adoption of GnRH antagonist cycles [1], the use of GnRH agonist triggers [2], the widespread availability of vitrification [3], the elective freeze-all policies [4], and the transition from fresh to remote frozen embryo transfer [5].

While numerous stimulation protocols have emerged recently to reduce OHSS—ranging from progesterone- and estrogen-primed protocols [6, 7] to the use of letrozole [8], metformin [9], inositol [10], dopamine agonists [11], and individualized gonadotropin dosing [12]—none offer the breadth of safety, efficacy, and cost-containment demonstrated by the IVF Lite protocol [13].

This chapter distills two decades of research and clinical progress into a single cohesive conclusion: that IVF Lite—when performed using mild stimulation, vitrification, preimplantation genetic testing for aneuploidy (PGTA), and remote transfer—fulfills the long-standing vision of an OHSS-free clinic [14]. Moreover, it offers a universally adaptable, biologically efficient model suited to a broad spectrum of patients, from hyper-responders to those with diminished ovarian reserve.

What follows is a synthesis of contemporary protocols proposed to prevent OHSS, leading up to the assertion that IVF Lite is not just an option—but the gold standard protocol for 2025.

18.2 Comparative Stimulation Strategies (2019–2025)

Recently, the quest for an ideal stimulation protocol that minimizes or eliminates the risk of ovarian hyperstimulation syndrome (OHSS) has led to a proliferation of strategies tailored to different patient phenotypes. Each protocol emerged in response to the growing consensus that OHSS is not merely manageable but preventable—especially when stimulation is individualized and embryo transfer is temporally uncoupled from follicular recruitment. This section critically evaluates the leading stimulation approaches proposed between 2019 and 2025, with a particular focus on their safety profiles and relevance in OHSS-prone populations.

1. *Progesterone-Primed Ovarian Stimulation (PPOS)* [15–17]

The PPOS protocol uses exogenous progestins in the follicular phase to suppress the luteinizing hormone (LH) surge, thereby replacing the need for GnRH antagonists. This approach allows cycle scheduling, simplifies patient management, and aligns well with freeze-all strategies. It has proven particularly useful in high responders and patients with PCOS, where premature LH surges and excessive follicular growth are primary concerns. Recent clinical data, including a 2025 consensus led by metformin [17], validate PPOS as an effective means to reduce early OHSS without compromising oocyte yield or embryo competence [18].

2. *Estrogen-Primed Protocols*

Estrogen priming, typically initiated in the luteal phase of the preceding cycle, synchronizes follicular cohorts by suppressing endogenous FSH. Its role is primarily in poor responders, where follicular asynchrony contributes to suboptimal stimulation. While physiological in concept and appealing in poor prognosis groups, the 2020 ESHRE guidelines stop short of recommending routine use due to limited conclusive evidence supporting its efficacy or safety in OHSS prevention [19]. Thus, estrogen priming remains an adjunctive tool, rather than a front-line solution.

3. *Letrozole-Augmented Stimulation*

Letrozole, an aromatase inhibitor, has gained traction as a minimal stimulation agent. By reducing systemic estradiol levels and enhancing endogenous gonadotropin secretion, it lowers the risk of OHSS while maintaining follicular responsiveness. Effective in

PCOS patients and those with estrogen-sensitive conditions, letrozole has been widely adopted in protocols where affordability and safety are paramount [8, 20].

While letrozole is not formally recognized as an OHSS prevention agent in major guidelines, multiple randomized trials and meta-analyses support its safety and efficacy when used in combination with low-dose gonadotropins [20, 21].

4. *Metformin Co-treatment*

Metformin continues to be prescribed in women with PCOS to address insulin resistance, improve ovulation, and reduce hyperandrogenism. Its proposed mechanism in OHSS prevention lies in its ability to reduce serum VEGF levels and suppress exaggerated follicular responses. However, as detailed in the HERA study, its effectiveness varies by protocol [22]. While early studies demonstrated clear benefits in GnRH agonist cycles, its efficacy in antagonist cycles has been questioned [22]. A Cochrane review concluded that although metformin reduces OHSS incidence, its impact on live birth remains inconclusive [23].

The most recent guidelines, therefore, suggest its use be limited to PCOS patients who are insulin-resistant, rather than applied universally for OHSS prevention [22, 23].

5. *Inositol Supplementation*

Inositol, particularly myoinositol and D-chiro-inositol, has been increasingly studied as a metabolic modulator in PCOS patients. It functions as a second messenger in insulin signaling and has been shown to improve ovulatory function and reduce oxidative stress. A 2024 RCT comparing myoinositol with metformin found comparable OHSS risk reduction, with fewer gastrointestinal side effects in the inositol arm [10]. However, other RCTs have flagged the overall quality of evidence as low [24, 25]. As of 2025, inositol remains an investigational adjunct with promise, but not yet a universally endorsed tool for OHSS prevention.

6. *Dopaminergic Agents*

Dopamine agonists such as cabergoline and quinagolide reduce OHSS risk by inhibiting VEGFR2-mediated vascular permeability. These agents are typically administered immediately after oocyte retrieval in high-risk patients. A 2021 Cochrane review confirmed a significant reduction in moderate-to-severe OHSS incidence with cabergoline, with no adverse impact on implantation or pregnancy rates [26].

Dopaminergic agents represent one of the most effective pharmacologic secondary preventives, especially in patients who are inadvertently overstimulated or exhibit borderline estradiol levels on trigger day. They are routinely combined with coasting or freeze-all strategies in risk mitigation protocols.

7. *Follitropin Delta (Individualized rFSH)*

Follitropin delta, a novel recombinant FSH, enables individualized dosing based on AMH levels and body weight. Four landmark studies published between 2021 and 2024 demonstrate significantly reduced early OHSS rates compared to conventional follitropin alfa, with comparable or superior live birth rates in normo- and high responders [27–30].

Despite its clinical appeal, the high cost, lack of cumulative outcome data, and limited accessibility in low-resource settings constrain its widespread adoption. Nevertheless, follitropin delta represents an evolution toward algorithm-driven, precision stimulation—an approach that aligns conceptually with the IVF Lite protocol.

18.3 IVF Lite: The Ideal Protocol in 2025

In the evolution of controlled ovarian stimulation, few protocols have achieved the convergence of safety, efficacy, accessibility, and biological efficiency that characterizes IVF Lite. As of 2025, it stands as the definitive stimulation protocol in the quest for an

OHSS-free clinic—not merely as an alternative for selected cases, but as a universal foundation adaptable to nearly every phenotype of ART patient [31].

The IVF Lite protocol is built on a core principle: mild stimulation, using oral ovulogens such as clomiphene citrate, with or without low-dose gonadotropins (typically 60–100 IU of FSH daily) [32]. This approach recruits a small, high-quality cohort of follicles while maintaining physiologic estradiol levels, drastically reducing the risk of VEGF-mediated capillary permeability—one of the central pathophysiologic mechanisms of OHSS. The goal is not to retrieve 15–20 oocytes, but to optimize the quality of 4–8 oocytes, most of which are mature, developmentally competent, and suitable for extended culture [31, 32].

Following oocyte retrieval, embryos are cultured to the blastocyst stage. At this point, the protocol is flexible: the blastocysts may either be vitrified directly or biopsied for preimplantation genetic testing for aneuploidy (PGTA) prior to cryopreservation. By eliminating the need for a fresh embryo transfer, IVF Lite fully decouples follicular stimulation from the luteal phase, eradicating the hormonal cascade responsible for early and late-onset OHSS [33]. The embryo transfer occurs in a remote frozen cycle, either hormonally prepared (HRT) or timed to a natural ovulatory cycle, depending on the patient's ovulatory status and clinical convenience.

What makes IVF Lite uniquely suited to the modern ART era is its broad-spectrum applicability. It is effective not only in patients traditionally considered ideal for minimal stimulation—such as women with low ovarian reserve or advanced maternal age—but also in groups that have historically posed the greatest risk for OHSS, including women with PCOS, hyper-responders, and those with a high antral follicle count [33]. In these populations, the use of clomiphene in place of (or prior to) gonadotropins results in controlled follicular development without the supraphysiologic estradiol spikes that characterize conventional protocols.

In patients with low AMH or diminished ovarian reserve, multiple IVF Lite cycles can be performed sequentially, with accumulation of vitrified blastocysts across time [31–33]. This "embryo banking" approach permits the eventual selection and transfer of a single euploid embryo, even in women with borderline ovarian function, while avoiding the physiologic stress of repeated high-dose stimulation. In older women, this strategy is particularly valuable, as it maximizes the probability of finding a chromosomally normal embryo without exposing the patient to unnecessary pharmacologic risk.

The cost-effectiveness of IVF Lite cannot be overstated. By drastically reducing the dose and duration of injectable medications and relying on oral agents for a significant portion of the cycle, the financial burden of ART becomes substantially more manageable—particularly in resource-constrained settings where affordability limits access. At the same time, the clinical pregnancy rates and live birth outcomes rival those of conventional stimulation, particularly when PGTA is employed to optimize embryo selection [34].

From a patient experience perspective, IVF Lite offers numerous advantages: fewer injections, minimal risk of OHSS, shorter monitoring visits, and flexibility in the timing of transfer. For clinicians, it delivers consistency, predictability, and a sharp reduction in cycle cancellations due to hyper-response.

Finally, IVF Lite is not a theoretical construct; it is a data-supported clinical pathway, with published outcomes demonstrating high implantation and pregnancy rates even in "difficult" patient cohorts. Its performance has been validated across diverse practice settings and patient demographics. It is a protocol grounded in biological plausibility, guided by the principles of patient safety, and refined by more than a decade of real-world use.

In 2025, IVF Lite is no longer a "mild" protocol. It is the protocol—for the patient, the clinician, and the clinic that aspires to eliminate OHSS completely.

18.4 Mild Stimulation Protocols Developed at Rotunda–CHR and Allahbadia IVF (2009–2025)

While IVF Lite has gained international traction in recent years, many of its foundational elements were conceptualized and systematically refined over nearly two decades at Rotunda—The Center For Human Reproduction, Mumbai, India (2009–2024) [5, 13, 31, 34] and further evolved at Allahbadia IVF, Dubai (2024–2025). These centers have been global pioneers in the development and clinical validation of mild ovarian stimulation protocols that prioritize safety, accessibility, and biological efficiency, with OHSS prevention as the non-negotiable cornerstone.

The common thread across all protocols developed in these programs is the universal use of GnRH antagonist cycles, enabling flexibility, LH surge suppression, and safe agonist triggering. These cycles consistently incorporate clomiphene citrate (commonly 50–100 mg/day) either as a standalone oral agent or in combination with low-dose gonadotropins (typically 60–100 IU/day of recombinant FSH or HMG), minimizing both cost and follicular over-response.

The evolution of these protocols was driven by three core objectives:

(a) To avoid OHSS across all patient types, including PCOS, hyper-responders, and younger women with high AFC or AMH levels.
(b) To reduce cost and injection burden, making ART accessible to patients in low-resource settings.
(c) To improve egg quality by avoiding excessive follicular recruitment and the hormonal imbalances that follow.

18.4.1 Among the most widely used protocols developed at these centers are

In all versions, the protocol culminates in a GnRH agonist trigger, blastocyst vitrification, with embryo pooling, with or without

PGTA and remote single embryo transfer—aligning with the structural design of IVF Lite. The use of antagonists as the foundational suppression strategy ensures cycle safety and minimizes luteal-phase complications, thereby reinforcing the OHSS-free framework.

These India- and UAE-based contributions to the global ART community have not only demonstrated clinical efficacy but also shown that protocol excellence does not require expensive pharmacology or complex infrastructure. What it requires is clarity of objective—OHSS elimination—and protocol discipline rooted in real-world feasibility.

18.4.2 Protocol 1: Clomiphene Citrate-Only Antagonist Cycle (Fig. 18.1)

This foundational mild stimulation protocol is designed for younger patients with PCOS or high ovarian reserve, where gonadotropin-free cycles are both biologically effective and economically preferable. The cycle begins with clomiphene citrate 100 mg daily from day 2 till follicular size reaches 22–23 mm, with no concurrent exogenous gonadotropins. Ultrasound moni-

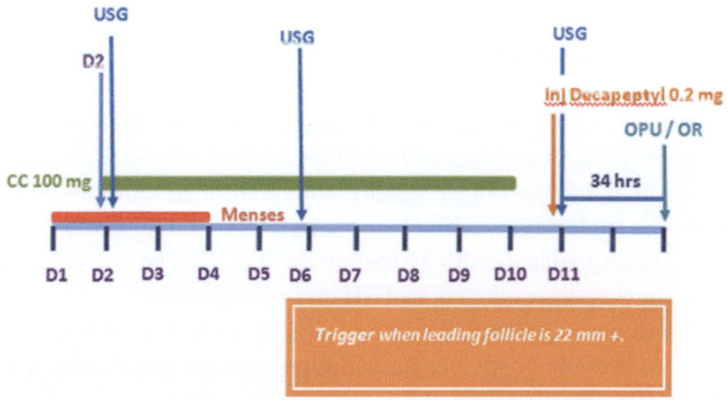

Fig. 18.1 Clomiphene-only antagonist protocols for young PCOS patients or those with financial constraints

toring is performed on days 2, 6, and 11, with adjustments in cycle timing based on follicular growth kinetics.

Luteinizing hormone (LH) surge suppression is achieved using a single 0.2 mg dose of leuprolide acetate (inj. decapeptyl) once the leading follicle reaches a mean diameter of ≥20 mm. Ovulation trigger is given at 22–23 mm average follicle size, followed by oocyte retrieval (OPU) 34 h later.

This protocol minimizes the risk of OHSS by avoiding supraphysiologic estradiol levels while maintaining high rates of follicular maturation.

It is especially suitable for:

- Cost-sensitive groups
- PCOS patients prone to hyper-response
- Clinics prioritizing OHSS-free cycles without gonadotropin use

Despite its simplicity, this protocol consistently yields competent oocytes and high-quality blastocysts when followed by vitrification and accumulation of biopsied or nonbiopsied blastocysts and deferred single embryo transfer.

18.4.3 Protocol 2: Clomiphene Plus Daily Low-Dose Gonadotropin with Antagonist Cover (Fig. 18.2)

This dual-agent stimulation protocol is ideal for poor responders, older women, or patients undergoing embryo banking for PGTA, where maximizing oocyte quality with controlled recruitment is key. The cycle begins with clomiphene citrate 100 mg daily from day 2 to follicular size 20–21 mm, initiating follicular recruitment while preserving endogenous FSH and LH dynamics.

From day 6 onward, menotropin (HMG) 75 IU is introduced daily to provide gentle exogenous support to the developing follicles. This combination enhances follicular maturation without pushing estradiol levels into the OHSS-risk zone.

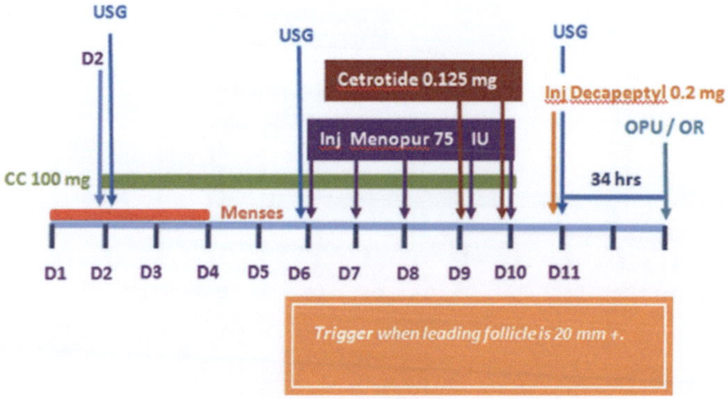

Fig. 18.2 Clomiphene +75 IU daily gonadotropin protocols for poor responders and DOR patients

To suppress the LH surge, cetrotide 0.125 mg is added from day 8 or 9, depending on follicular response. Ovulation is triggered using a GnRH agonist (decapeptyl 0.2 mg) once the leading follicle reaches 20–21 mm, followed by oocyte retrieval 34 h later.

This protocol provides:

- A balance of oral and injectable agents for cost containment
- Effective stimulation in low-AMH or advanced age groups
- Minimal OHSS risk due to physiologic estrogen levels and antagonist control
- It is particularly useful in repeat IVF attempts and PGTA cycles. Clinical results at both Rotunda–CHR and Allahbadia IVF have demonstrated consistent oocyte maturity, high-quality blastocyst development, and good euploidy rate using this approach.

18.4.4 Protocol 3: Clomiphene with Alternate-Day Gonadotropin and Antagonist Cover (Fig. 18.3)

This protocol reflects a strategic refinement of mild stimulation, designed to further reduce gonadotropin burden and treatment cost without compromising follicular quality. It is ideal for

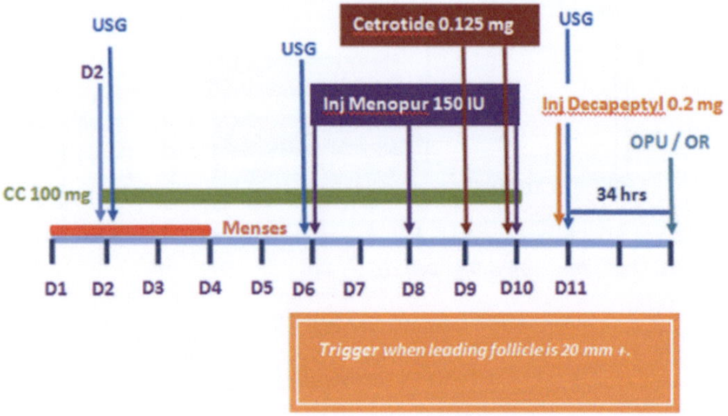

Fig. 18.3 Clomiphene +150 IU daily gonadotropin alternate day protocols for poor responders and DOR patients

cost-sensitive patients, including those undergoing IVF Lite or embryo pooling cycles.

Stimulation begins with clomiphene citrate 100 mg daily from days 2 to 10, supporting early follicular recruitment. Menotropin 150 IU is administered on alternate days—typically on days 6, 8, and 10—targeting follicular support only during critical growth windows. This structured spacing minimizes total gonadotropin exposure while maintaining sufficient estradiol production for optimal folliculogenesis.

To prevent premature LH surge, cetrotide 0.125 mg is initiated from day 8 or 9, depending on lead follicle size and estradiol trends. Ovulation is triggered using decapeptyl 0.2 mg when the leading follicle reaches 20–21 mm, followed by oocyte retrieval 34 h later.

This protocol is especially suited for:

- Patients in remote or satellite cycle programs.
- Those requiring a balance between affordability and oocyte yield.
- Clinics with limited gonadotropin availability.

Its alternate-day design ensures biologically timed gonadotropin exposure while avoiding hormonal excess. Data from Rotunda–CHR and Allahbadia IVF confirm that this protocol delivers consistent blastocyst quality, good euploidy rates, and low complication rates—making it a resource-efficient, OHSS-safe strategy for modern ART.

18.4.5 Protocol 4: Low-Dose Daily Gonadotropin Antagonist Cycle (Fig. 18.4)

This protocol is optimized for patients with diminished ovarian reserve (DOR), advanced maternal age, or those with repeated implantation failure who may benefit from improved follicular output without overstimulation. Daily recombinant FSH or HMG (60–100 IU) is initiated from day 51/2, continuing till follicular size reaches 19–20 mm. The stimulation aims to support a focused follicular cohort while avoiding multifollicular response and excessive estradiol rise.

Transvaginal ultrasounds are performed on days 2, 6, and 9 to monitor follicular progression. A GnRH antagonist (cetrotide 0.125 mg) is introduced from day 8 or 9 onwards for LH surge suppression once follicles begin to approach preovulatory size.

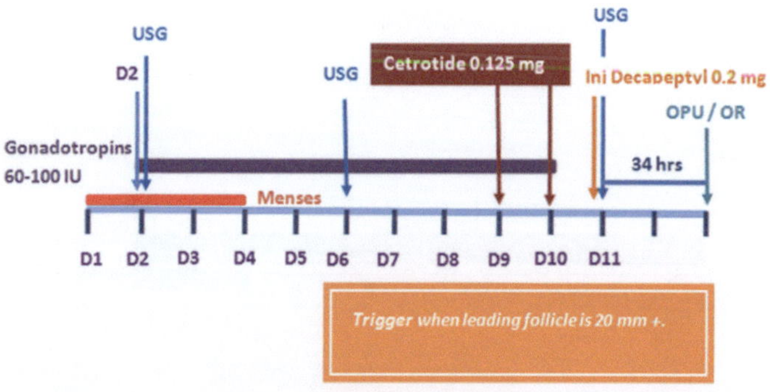

Fig. 18.4 Low-dose gonadotropin protocols for all indications (60–100 IU mHG or recFSH)

Ovulation is triggered using a GnRH agonist (inj. Decapeptyl 0.2 mg) when the leading follicle reaches 19–20 mm, and oocyte retrieval is timed 34 h later.

This low-dose antagonist protocol is especially effective in:

Older women seeking embryo accumulation cycles

Patients undergoing IVF Lite with blastocyst vitrification

Situations where PGTA is planned, but hyper-response must be avoided

It balances follicular recruitment with maintaining a strong safety profile and low OHSS risk. The mild gonadotropin exposure ensures that retrieved oocytes have optimal cytoplasmic maturity without the dysregulation often seen in conventional high-dose regimens.

18.4.6 Protocol 5: Elonva One Protocol (Fig. 18.5)

The Elonva One Protocol is a streamlined mild stimulation approach that leverages a single injection of corifollitropin alfa (Elonva 150 mcg) to provide extended FSH activity across the early follicular phase, paired with clomiphene citrate to optimize follicular recruitment. This protocol is ideal for a broad spectrum of patients, including those with low AMH, diminished ovarian

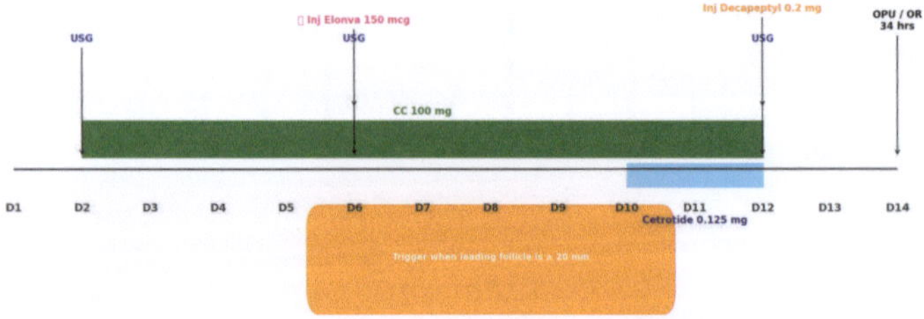

Fig. 18.5 Elonva One protocol with clomiphene and 150 ug corifollitropin alpha for poor responders and DOR patients

reserve (DOR), older age, and cost constraints—but not for hyper-responders or PCOS patients, due to the risk of overstimulation.

The protocol begins with clomiphene citrate 100 mg daily from day 1/2 till follicular size 20–21 mm. A single dose of Elonva 150 mcg is administered on day 5/6, replacing the need for daily gonadotropin injections for the following 7 days. GnRH antagonist coverage (cetrotide 0.125 mg) is introduced at follicular size 18–19 mm to prevent premature LH surge.

Triggering is performed with decapeptyl 0.2 mg, and oocyte retrieval is scheduled 34 h later. Ultrasound monitoring is conducted on days 2, 6, 9, and 11, with the trigger administered when the leading follicle reaches ≥20 mm.

This protocol offers several advantages:

- Patient convenience with fewer injections
- Cost-effectiveness through minimal gonadotropin use
- Strong end-organ response in normo-responders and older patients
- Full compatibility with OHSS-free, freeze-all strategies
- It integrates seamlessly into IVF Lite and embryo pooling protocols where safety, simplicity, and efficiency are paramount.

18.4.7 Protocol 6: Elonva Two Protocol (Fig. 18.6)

The Elonva Two Protocol offers a highly simplified, patient friendly ovarian stimulation strategy suitable for normo responders, older women, and those with diminished ovarian reserve (DOR). It is not intended for hyper-responders or PCOS

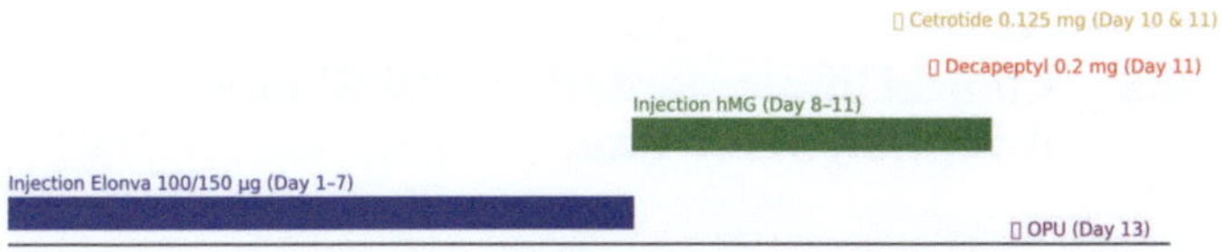

Fig. 18.6 Elonva Two protocol with 100 or 150 ug corifollitropin alpha for poor responders and DOR patients

patients due to the sustained gonadotropic action of corifollitropin alfa. This protocol is distinguished by its minimal injection requirement and its compatibility with OHSS-free, freeze-all IVF workflows.

Stimulation begins with a single subcutaneous injection of inj. Elonva, administered on day 1 or 2, with the dose determined by patient weight: 100 mcg for those under 60 kg and 150 mcg for those above 60 kg. This long-acting recombinant FSH analogue provides effective follicular stimulation for up to 7 days, eliminating the need for daily gonadotropin injections during the early follicular phase. From day 8, we give 75 IU hMG till follicular size 20–21 mm.

Monitoring with transvaginal ultrasound is performed on days 2, 6, 9, and 11. Once the leading follicle reaches 18–19 mm, GnRH antagonist coverage with cetrotide 0.125 mg is initiated to prevent premature LH surge. Ovulation trigger is given using decapeptyl 0.2 mg, and oocyte retrieval (OPU/OR) is performed 34 h later. The protocol is designed to trigger once the leading follicle reaches 20–21 mm, optimizing oocyte maturity while maintaining a low estrogen environment.

This protocol is particularly useful for:

- Women with low ovarian reserve who prefer minimal injections
- Patients undergoing IVF Lite or embryo banking cycles
- Clinics implementing simplified stimulation models without compromising outcomes
- When combined with blastocyst vitrification and deferred single embryo transfer, the Elonva Two Protocol supports both clinical efficacy and OHSS prevention.

18.5 Clinical Implementation and Global Adoption of IVF Lite

The real-world success of any medical protocol lies not only in its theoretical superiority but also in its reproducibility, adaptability, and impact across clinical settings. IVF Lite has steadily transitioned from a niche alternative to a globally recognized and implemented standard of care in OHSS-free ART practice. As of 2025, its incorporation into mainstream clinical algorithms is evidence not only of its safety but also of its superior strategic alignment with the evolution of IVF into a safer, more patient-centered, and biologically rational discipline.

18.5.1 A Protocol Adapted to Diverse Populations

The versatility of IVF Lite lies in its modularity. The core concept—mild stimulation followed by freeze-all—can be adapted across varied patient profiles and geographic contexts. In high-resource centers, IVF Lite has been adopted with comprehensive PGTA, allowing the identification and deferred transfer of a single euploid embryo with high implantation potential [33]. In low- and middle-income settings, where cost and access to daily injections can be prohibitive, the use of clomiphene citrate with minimal gonadotropins significantly lowers treatment barriers while preserving clinical outcomes.

Women with polycystic ovary syndrome (PCOS), historically at the highest risk of developing OHSS, benefit enormously from the physiology-preserving stimulation inherent to IVF Lite. Unlike conventional antagonist cycles that rely on high-dose gonadotropins and risk dose overshooting, IVF Lite's strategy of clomiphene or letrozole priming allows follicular recruitment in a controlled, steady fashion, leading to a lower number of retrieved oocytes—but with consistently high maturation and blastocyst development rates.

For hyper-responders, including those with elevated AMH or high AFC, the protocol's ceiling on gonadotropin stimulation serves as a built-in safety mechanism. Unlike high-dose regimens, which may result in cycle cancellation or coasting, IVF Lite circumvents the risk of triggering an exaggerated VEGF cascade and thereby eliminates the root of OHSS pathogenesis.

In older patients and those with diminished ovarian reserve (DOR), IVF Lite is equally relevant. In this cohort, repeated high-dose stimulation is not only unnecessary but also biologically unproductive. Instead, sequential mild stimulation cycles with embryo pooling enable a practical path to euploid embryo transfer, often increasing cumulative success rates without the physiologic burden of repeated high-intensity cycles.

At clinics such as Allahbadia IVF, for instance, patients undergo ovarian stimulation and oocyte retrieval in Dubai, followed by vitrification and PGTA, with the euploid embryo transferred months later in a hormone-prepped cycle. This model leverages IVF Lite's segmentation to offer flexibility, patient compliance, and time-optimized care.

18.5.2 Reproducibility and Training

IVF Lite's appeal also lies in its reproducibility. It is easily taught, protocolized, and executed across centers. Unlike advanced stimulation regimens requiring individualized daily titrations and extensive monitoring, IVF Lite's core structure is elegant in its simplicity. Most protocols follow a 12–14-day cycle with minimal dose modifications and predictable hormonal profiles. This makes it ideal for scaling across national ART networks, as well as for training programs looking to standardize safe, effective IVF care.

18.5.3 Remote-Cycle Workflows and In-clinic Embryo Accumulation with PGTA

The clinic follows a rigorously structured model of:

Accumulating biopsied vitrified blastocysts over one or more stimulation cycles

Freezing the biopsied trophectoderm cells in a designated freezer until the target number of embryos is reached

Once the cohort is complete, all biopsies are sent simultaneously for PGTA using next-generation sequencing (NGS)

Only euploid embryos are retained in cryostorage, while aneuploid embryos are discarded in accordance with clinic policy
A single euploid embryo is later transferred in an estrogen-primed HRT replacement cycle, typically in a remote visit

This strategy enables patients—including those with low AMH, poor ovarian reserve, or previous IVF failures—to achieve high pregnancy outcomes without risking OHSS or undergoing high-intensity stimulation.

At Allahbadia IVF, this approach consistently delivers clinical pregnancy rates exceeding 60%, even in traditionally poor-prognosis groups. The protocol represents the full operationalization of IVF Lite as an OHSS-free, biologically rational, and legally compliant ART strategy.

18.6 Global Data and Outcomes

Clinical studies and retrospective cohort analyses from India, Japan, and the United States have consistently shown that minimal stimulation IVF and remote transfers of vitrified embryos produce high-quality blastocysts, maintain cumulative live birth rates comparable to conventional IVF, and reduce both medication cost and cycle complications. A series of studies from centers in India and abroad—including those authored by Allahbadia and colleagues over the past two decades—have been foundational in establishing the role of clomiphene-based minimal stimulation with freeze-all and remote transfer in modern ART [34–37].

With over a decade of safety data and thousands of cycles performed worldwide, IVF Lite is no longer experimental or supplementary—it is an established protocol. Its global adoption reflects not only a shift in clinical preference but also a deeper realignment of reproductive medicine toward biologic plausibility, patient safety, and outcome optimization.

18.7 The Future of Stimulation: IVF Lite as the Algorithmic Endpoint

The history of ovarian stimulation in assisted reproduction has moved from aggressive gonadotropin regimens focused on oocyte yield toward a new paradigm: personalized, physiologic, and OHSS-free stimulation. As of 2025, this evolution reaches its most rational and biologically aligned expression in IVF Lite—a strategy no longer "mild," but mainstream.

IVF Lite embodies every advancement the field has made in the last two decades: the use of oral ovulogens, antagonist suppression, agonist triggers, vitrification, PGTA, and remote-cycle segmentation. Together, these elements form a cohesive protocol that minimizes risk while maintaining efficacy across nearly all patient phenotypes.

Unlike conventional stimulation, IVF Lite does not attempt to over-recruit follicles or push supraphysiologic estradiol levels. Instead, it maximizes the developmental potential of a smaller, higher-quality cohort of oocytes. By focusing on euploidy rather than quantity, and by separating the stimulation and transfer phases, the protocol prevents both early and late-onset OHSS. As practiced at centers like Allahbadia IVF, Dubai, IVF Lite achieves >60% pregnancy rates in even poor prognosis patients, with virtually zero incidence of OHSS.

The incorporation of PGTA via NGS, single euploid embryo transfer, and HRT-based remote cycle preparation has enabled this model to be both globally adaptable and scientifically grounded. With strict policies on discarding aneuploid embryos and freezing only chromosomally normal blastocysts, IVF Lite now functions not only as a treatment protocol but also as an algorithmic standard for modern ART.

As artificial intelligence and predictive modeling continue to shape individualized medicine, IVF Lite is uniquely positioned to integrate algorithm-driven dose modulation, stimulation personalization, and embryo selection. It is not a stepping stone toward future protocols—it is the destination.

Clinics and programs aiming to modernize, simplify, and completely eliminate the risk of OHSS will find in IVF Lite a framework that is evidence-based, scalable, and patient-centric.

References

1. Papanikolaou EG, et al. Preventing OHSS: gonadotropin-releasing hormone antagonist protocols. Reprod Biomed Online. 2005;10(4):335–45. PMID: 15901484.
2. Delvigne A, Rozenberg S. Review of clinical course and treatment of ovarian hyperstimulation syndrome (OHSS). Hum Reprod Update. 2003;9(1):77–96. PMID: 12519319.
3. Aboulghar MA. Prevention of OHSS. Reprod Biomed Online. 2009;19(1):33–42. PMID: 19549483.
4. Allahbadia GN. Getting older women pregnant: contemporary thoughts. J Obstet Gynaecol India. 2016;66(5):305–9. https://doi.org/10.1007/s13224-015-0804-8. Epub 2015 Nov 13. PMID: 27486273; PMCID: PMC4958080.
5. Allahbadia GN. The ideal stimulation protocol: is there one? J Obstet Gynaecol India. 2015;65(6):357–61. https://doi.org/10.1007/s13224-015-0723-8. Epub 2015 Jul 1. PMID: 26663992; PMCID: PMC4666208.
6. Kalafat E, Turkgeldi E, Yıldız S, Dizdar M, Keles I, Ata B. Outcomes of a GnRH agonist trigger following a GnRH antagonist or flexible progestin-primed ovarian stimulation. Cycle.Front Endocrinol (Lausanne). 2022;13:837880. https://doi.org/10.3389/fendo.2022.837880. eCollection 2022.
7. Ceyhan T, Ozturk M, Yıldız UG, Fidan U, Agacayak E, Ulubay M, Korkmaz C. Repeated application of luteal phase oestradiol/GnRH antagonist priming increases IVF success for poor ovarian reserve patients. J Obstet Gynaecol. 2023;43(2):2211664. https://doi.org/10.1080/01443615.2023.2211664.
8. Jiang L, Qiu Y, Xu L, et al. Aromatase inhibitors to prevent OHSS in IVF: a systematic review and meta-analysis. Reprod Biol Endocrinol. 2024;22(1):85. https://doi.org/10.1186/s12958-024-01258-y. PMID: 39044268; PMCID: PMC11265326.
9. Andavar M, Kamaraj R, Vijayakumar TM, et al. Dual therapy of acarbose with metformin or myo-inositol in PCOS: RCT. Eur J Obstet Gynecol Reprod Biol. 2024;300:6–11. https://doi.org/10.1016/j.ejogrb.2024.07.001.

10. Lin L, Chen G, Qiao X, Chen Y, Deng H, Xu L. Comparative efficacy and safety of metformin, anti-obesity agents, and myoinositol in improving IVF/ICSI outcomes and reducing ovarian hyperstimulation syndrome in women with polycystic ovary syndrome: a systematic review and network meta-analysis. J Ovarian Res. 2024;17(1):249. https://doi.org/10.1186/s13048-024-01576-0.
11. Baradwan S, AlJaroudi D, Agdi M, Hafedh B, Abduljabbar HH, Sabban H, Alzawawi N, Alsaad N, Alshahrani MS, Idriss A, AlSghan R, Asiri M, Baradwan A, Edrees A, Abu-Zaid A. Calcium versus cabergoline for prevention of ovarian hyperstimulation syndrome: a systematic review and meta-analysis. Eur J Obstet Gynecol Reprod Biol. 2024;301:1–11. https://doi.org/10.1016/j.ejogrb.2024.07.054. Epub 2024 Jul 27.
12. Weiss NS, Kostova EB, Mol BWJ, van Wely M. Gonadotropins for ovulation induction in women with PCOS. Cochrane Database Syst Rev. 2025;4(4):CD010290. https://doi.org/10.1002/14651858.CD010290.pub4. PMID: 40193219; PMCID: PMC11975188.
13. Allahbadia GN. IVF lite: is this the future of assisted reproduction? J Obstet Gynaecol India. 2013;63(1):1–4. https://doi.org/10.1007/s13224-013-0402-6. PMID: 24431590; PMCID: PMC3650145.
14. Gianaroli L, Vitagliano A, Ferraretti AP, Azzena S, Terzuoli G, Perruzza D, Ambrosini G, Tabanelli C, Magli MC. IVF Lite: a smart IVF programme based on mild ovarian stimulation for good prognosis patients. Reprod Biomed Online. 2022;45(2):256–63. https://doi.org/10.1016/j.rbmo.2022.04.003. Epub 2022 Apr 14.
15. Guan S, Feng Y, Huang Y, Huang J. Progestin-primed ovarian stimulation protocol for patients in assisted reproductive technology: a meta-analysis of randomized controlled trials. Front Endocrinol (Lausanne). 2021;12:702558. https://doi.org/10.3389/fendo.2021.702558. eCollection 2021.
16. Dong M, Sun L, Huang L, Wang F, Zhang X, Liu F. Fixed gonadotropin-releasing hormone antagonist protocol versus flexible progestin-primed ovarian stimulation protocol in patients with asynchronous follicular development during controlled ovulation stimulation: a retrospective study. Front Endocrinol (Lausanne). 2021;12:690575. https://doi.org/10.3389/fendo.2021.690575. eCollection 2021.
17. Leathersich S, Roche C, Hart R. Minimising OHSS in women with PCOS. Front Endocrinol (Lausanne). 2025;16:1507857. https://doi.org/10.3389/fendo.2025.1507857. PMID: 40182629; PMCID: PMC11966453.
18. Souza MM, Souza MDCB, Antunes RA, Barbeitas AL, Raupp VA, Souza ALBM, Silva LABD, Mancebo ACA, Sequeira FF. Dydrogesterone is an eligible tool to suppress LH surge in assisted reproduction technologies (ART) cycles. JBRA Assist Reprod. 2025; https://doi.org/10.5935/1518-0557.20250003. Online ahead of print.

19. Ovarian Stimulation TEGGO, Bosch E, Broer S, Griesinger G, Grynberg M, Humaidan P, Kolibianakis E, Kunicki M, La Marca A, Lainas G, Le Clef N, Massin N, Mastenbroek S, Polyzos N, Sunkara SK, Timeva T, Töyli M, Urbancsek J, Vermeulen N, Broekmans F. ESHRE guideline: ovarian stimulation for IVF/ICSI†. Hum Reprod Open. 2020;2020(2):hoaa009. https://doi.org/10.1093/hropen/hoaa009. Erratum in: Hum Reprod Open. 2020 Dec 29;2020(4):hoaa067. https://doi.org/10.1093/hropen/hoaa067. PMID: 32395637; PMCID: PMC7203749.
20. Li J, Peng Y, Dai X, Zhang L, Long X, Wang X, Li W, Fang Y, Xiong W, Liu Y. Human menopausal gonadotropin (HMG) combined different doses of letrozole for treating anovulatory infertility in patients with polycystic ovary syndrome: a randomized controlled trial. J Assist Reprod Genet. 2025; https://doi.org/10.1007/s10815-025-03455-z. Epub ahead of print.
21. Jiang L, Qiu Y, Xu L, Chang R, He F. Effect of aromatase inhibitors for preventing ovarian hyperstimulation syndrome in infertile patients undergoing in vitro fertilization: a systematic review and meta-analysis. Reprod Biol Endocrinol. 2024;22(1):85. https://doi.org/10.1186/s12958-024-01258-y. PMID: 39044268; PMCID: PMC11265326.
22. Feferkorn I, Santos-Ribeiro S, Ubaldi FM, Velasco JG, Ata B, Blockeel C, Conforti A, Esteves SC, Fatemi HM, Gianaroli L, Grynberg M, Humaidan P, Lainas GT, La Marca A, Craig LB, Lathi R, Norman RJ, Orvieto R, Paulson R, Pellicer A, Polyzos NP, Roque M, Sunkara SK, Tan SL, Urman B, Venetis C, Weissman A, Yarali H, Dahan MH. The HERA (Hyper-response Risk Assessment) Delphi consensus for the management of hyper-responders in in vitro fertilization. J Assist Reprod Genet. 2023;40(11):2681–95. https://doi.org/10.1007/s10815-023-02918-5. Epub 2023 Sep 15. Erratum in: J Assist Reprod Genet. 2024 Feb;41(2):519–520. https://doi.org/10.1007/s10815-023-03003-7. PMID: 37713144; PMCID: PMC10643792.
23. Mourad S, Brown J, Farquhar C. Interventions for the prevention of OHSS in ART cycles: an overview of Cochrane reviews. Cochrane Database Syst Rev. 2017;1(1):CD012103. https://doi.org/10.1002/14651858.CD012103.pub2. PMID: 28111738; PMCID: PMC6469542.
24. Rajasekaran K, Malhotra N, Mahey R, Khadgawat R, Kalaivani M. Myoinositol versus metformin pretreatment in GnRH-antagonist cycle for women with PCOS undergoing IVF: a double-blinded randomized controlled study. Gynecol Endocrinol. 2022;38(2):140–7. https://doi.org/10.1080/09513590.2021.1981282. Epub 2021 Sep 30.
25. Agrawal A, Mahey R, Kachhawa G, Khadgawat R, Vanamail P, Kriplani A. Comparison of metformin plus myoinositol vs metformin alone in PCOS women undergoing ovulation induction cycles: randomized controlled trial. Gynecol Endocrinol. 2019;35(6):511–4. https://doi.org/10.1080/09513590.2018.1549656. Epub 2019 Jan 7.

26. Tang H, Mourad SM, Wang A, Zhai SD, Hart RJ. Dopamine agonists for preventing ovarian hyperstimulation syndrome. Cochrane Database Syst Rev. 2021;4(4):CD008605. https://doi.org/10.1002/14651858.CD008605.pub4. PMID: 33851429; PMCID: PMC8092425.
27. Lobo R, Soerdal T, Ekerhovd E, Cohlen B, Porcu E, Schenk M, Shufaro Y, Smeenk J, Suerdieck MB, Pinton P, Pinborg A, Investigators BEYOND. BEYOND: a randomized controlled trial comparing efficacy and safety of individualized follitropin delta dosing in a GnRH agonist versus antagonist protocol during the first ovarian stimulation cycle. Hum Reprod. 2024;39(7):1481–94. https://doi.org/10.1093/humrep/deae092. Epub ahead of print. PMID: 38723189; PMCID: PMC11759129.
28. Komiya S, Watanabe J, Terayama T, Kamijo K, Okada H. Efficacy and safety of follitropin delta versus follitropin alpha/beta in infertility treatment: a systematic review and meta-analysis. Reprod Med Biol. 2024;23(1):e12573. https://doi.org/10.1002/rmb2.12573. PMID: 38528991; PMCID: PMC10961712.
29. Palomba S, Caserta D, Levi-Setti PE, Busnelli A. Efficacy and safety of follitropin delta for ovarian stimulation in vitro fertilization/intracytoplasmic sperm injection cycles: a systematic review with meta-analysis. J Ovarian Res. 2024;17(1):60. https://doi.org/10.1186/s13048-024-01372-w. PMID: 38486276; PMCID: PMC10938807.
30. Porcu-Buisson G, Maignien C, Swierkowski-Blanchard N, Rongières C, Ranisavljevic N, Oger P, Decanter C, Hocké C, Bry-Gauillard H, Grynberg M, Barrière P, Bernot M, Guivarc'h-Levêque A. Prospective multicenter observational real-world study to assess the use, efficacy and safety profile of follitropin delta during IVF/ICSI procedures (DELTA study). Eur J Obstet Gynecol Reprod Biol. 2024;293:21–6. https://doi.org/10.1016/j.ejogrb.2023.12.011. Epub 2023 Dec 9.
31. Allahbadia GN. Have we finally written the obituary for conventional IVF? ivflite. 2014;1:1–5. https://doi.org/10.4103/2348-2907.127081.
32. Bodri D, Kawachiya S, De Brucker M, Tournaye H, Kondo M, Kato R, Matsumoto T. Cumulative success rates following mild IVF in unselected infertile patients: a 3-year, single-centre cohort study. Reprod Biomed Online. 2014;28(5):572–81. https://doi.org/10.1016/j.rbmo.2014.01.002. Epub 2014 Jan 24.
33. Zhang J. Resurgence of minimal Stimulation in vitro fertilization with a protocol consisting of gonadotropin releasing hormone-agonist trigger and vitrified-thawed embryo transfer. Int J Fertil Steril. 2016;10(2):148–53. https://doi.org/10.22074/ijfs.2016.4903. Epub 2016 Jun 1.
34. Allahbadia GN. Stimulation and aneuploidy: why are milder stimulation protocols better? IVF Lite. 2016;3:41–5. https://doi.org/10.4103/2348-2907.192281.

35. Kato K, Kuroda T, Yamadera-Egawa R, Ezoe K, Aoyama N, Usami A, Miki T, Yamamoto T, Takeshita T. Preimplantation genetic testing for aneuploidy for recurrent pregnancy loss and recurrent implantation failure in minimal Ovarian Stimulation cycle for women aged 35-42 years: live birth rate, developmental follow-up of children, and embryo ranking. Reprod Sci. 2023;30(3):974–83. https://doi.org/10.1007/s43032-022-01073-z. Epub 2022 Sep 9.
36. Zhang JJ, Merhi Z, Yang M, Bodri D, Chavez-Badiola A, Repping S, van Wely M. Minimal stimulation IVF vs conventional IVF: a randomized controlled trial. Am J Obstet Gynecol. 2016;214(1):96.e1–8. https://doi.org/10.1016/j.ajog.2015.08.009. Epub 2015 Aug 8.
37. Kato K, Takehara Y, Segawa T, Kawachiya S, Okuno T, Kobayashi T, Bodri D, Kato O. Minimal ovarian stimulation combined with elective single embryo transfer policy: age-specific results of a large, single-centre, Japanese cohort. Reprod Biol Endocrinol. 2012;10:35. https://doi.org/10.1186/1477-7827-10-35.

MIX
Papier aus verantwortungsvollen Quellen
Paper from responsible sources
FSC® C105338
FSC
www.fsc.org

If you have any concerns about our products,
you can contact us on
ProductSafety@springernature.com

In case Publisher is established outside the EU,
the EU authorized representative is:
Springer Nature Customer Service Center GmbH
Europaplatz 3, 69115 Heidelberg, Germany

Printed by Libri Plureos GmbH
in Hamburg, Germany